AYUSH in Public Health

About the Author

Prof. R. K. Mutatkar, a student of Prof. S. C. Dube and a colleague of Prof. Irawati Karve was the first Head of the Department of Anthropology and the first Director of the School of Health Sciences, University of Pune. He pioneered teaching of Medical Anthropology in India in 1974. He initiated social science research on Leprosy at WHO, Geneva in 1981. He chaired the curriculum development committee for Anthropology at the UGC to prepare a model syllabus in 2001. He was Chairman of the first working group of AYUSH in Public Health at the Steering Committee on AYUSH for the XI Five Year Plan. He has been Chairman of the Indian National Confederation and Academy of Anthropologists (INCAA). He established an academic NGO, The Maharashtra Association of Anthropological Sciences, (MAAS) in 1976 at Pune.

Currently he is Chairman of the Scientific Advisory Group of the Social-Behavioural Research Division of the ICMR. Society for Indian Medical Anthropology (SIMA) organized a conference in his honour at Mysore in 2007 and dedicated two volumes "Explorations in Indian Medical Anthropology" to him, published by Concept Publishing Company Pvt. Ltd.

Prof. Mutatkar was honoured with International Gandhi Award for Leprosy, on 30th January, 2016, which is World Leprosy Day and Martyr's Day in India, by Hon. Vice President of India, Shri Hamid Ansari, at New Delhi.

AYUSH IN PUBLIC HEALTH

Volume One
Traditional Healthcare System

R.K. Mutatkar

Jointly Published
for
Centre: AYUSH in Public Health
The Maharashtra Association of Anthropological Sciences
(MAAS)
by

CONCEPT PUBLISHING COMPANY PVT. LTD.
NEW DELHI-110059

ISBN-13: 978-93-5125-228-3 (Set)
ISBN-13: 978-93-5125-229-0 (Vol. I)
ISBN-13: 978-93-5125-230-6 (Vol. II)

First Published 2016

Published and Printed by:

Concept
Since 1974

Concept Publishing Company Pvt. Ltd.
A/15-16, Commercial Block, Mohan Garden,
New Delhi-110059 (INDIA)
Phones : 25351460, 25351794, *Fax* : 091-11-25357109
E-mail : publishing@conceptpub.com
Website: www.conceptpub.com

Editorial Office: H-13, Bali Nagar, New Delhi-110 015, India.

Cataloging in Publication Data—DK Courtesy: D.K. Agencies (P) Ltd. <docinfo@dkagencies.com>

Mutatkar, R. K. (Ramchandra Keshav), 1936- **author.**

AYUSH in public health / R.K. Mutatkar
volumes cm

Contents: volume I. Traditional healthcare system — volume II. A handbook for research and training.

ISBN 9789351252283 (set)
ISBN 9789351252290 (vol. I)
ISBN 9789351252306 (vol. II)

1. Medical care—India. 2. Traditional medicine—Government policy—India. 3. Alternative medicine—Government policy—India. 4. Medical policy—India. 5. India. Department of Ayurveda, Yoga & Naturopathy, Unani, Siddha, and Homoeopathy. I. Mutatkar, Kalpana, author. II. India. Department of Ayurveda, Yoga & Naturopathy, Unani, Siddha, and Homoeopathy, publisher. III. Maharashtra Association of Anthropological Sciences, publisher. IV. Title.

RA529.M88 2016 DDC 362.10954 23

DEDICATION

The book is dedicated to the memory of the scholars who helped to develop AYUSH Public Health Perspectives in Medical Anthropology since the International Symposium on Medical Anthropology at Pune University in December 1978, by personal encouragement at every level.

1. Prof. Charles Leslie, eminent medical anthropologist from U.S. whose edited book 'Asian Medical Systems' is a classic reference volume. First Secretary-General, International Association for the Study of Traditional Asian Medicine (IASTAM), Canberra, 1979.
2. Vaidya Pandit Shiv Sharma, doyen of Ayurved in Independent India, who rejuvenated Indian Systems of Medicine by establishing and heading CCIM to propagate AYUSH medical education and therapy. First Vice President, IASTAM, Canberra, 1979, First President, IASTAM-India, 1980.
3. Prof. A.L. Basham: Eminent Indologist from Australia whose book 'The Wonder that was India' is unparalleled classic. Took initiative in the multidisciplinary studies of Traditional Asian Medicine by hosting first ICTAM in September 1979 at Canberra. First President, IASTAM.

But for the dedication and affection of these Pandits, AYUSH would not have been discussed as public health agenda, starting with Eleventh Five Year Plan. Studies on AYUSH in Indian Medical Anthropology are the direct outcome of their promotion.

VISION : NATIONAL AYUSH POLICY

"Ayurveda, Homoeopathy, Siddha, Unani, Yoga and Naturopathy offer a wide range of preventive, promotive and curative treatment that are both cost effective and efficacious. We are working to end the long neglect of these holistic systems in our national healthcare strategy. A National Medicinal Plant Board has been set up to promote cultivation, processing, production, and standaradization of herbal products, both for domestic and export markets. Steps are also being taken to protect our traditional knowledge in this area, which promised to attract immense global attention in the coming years."

Shri K. R. Narayanan
President of India
Address: Joint Session of Parliament
19th February, 2001

"In recent years, there has been a great interest, both in India and abroad, in Ayurveda and other Indian Systems of Medicine. We are considering making available a low-cost kit containing certain traditional medicines and herbal products, which have proved their efficacy over centuries in treating many common ailments. I urge our kisans and pharmaceutical companies to seize this new opportunity created by the growing worldwide attraction for Ayurvedic products and Indian systems of Medicine."

Shri Atal Bihari Vajpayee
Prime Minister of India
Independence Day Speech, 15th August, 2001

Maharashtra Association of Anthropological Sciences (MAAS)

Maharashtra Association of Anthropological Sciences (MAAS), was established at the University of Pune in 1976 as an academic NGO supported by the then Vice Chancellor, Principal D.A. Dabholkar. Developed as an open platform to bring together academics, activists, policy planners and administrators to discuss issues around tribal development, health, environment, gender, culture and education in the perspective of holistic human development. MAAS has been Asian partner of LSHTM for a decade focusing on operational research about T.B. and HIV. MAAS had an intervention project about tribal malnutrition from the State Government. Department of AYUSH, Government of India offered a project to assess ground level situation about AYUSH in four States of India, followed by awarding "Centre for AYUSH in Public Health" to develop as a Centre of Excellence.

Established by Prof. R.K. Mutatkar, MAAS had illustrious Presidents such as, an eminent Marathi Litterateur Prof. G.B. Sardar, President, Marathi Sahitya Sammelan; Sri Janardan Walvi, a Bhil educationist; Prof. P.V. Sukhatme, Padma Bhushan and Prof. A.R. Kulkarni, Chairman, ICHR, followed by Prof. R.K. Mutatkar who was founder General Secretary earlier. Current President of MAAS is Prof. S. Parasuraman, Director of Tata Institute of Social Sciences (TISS), an anthropologist-demographer who has succeeded Prof. P.B. Vidyasagar, Vice-Chancellor, Swami Ramanand Tirth Marathwada University, Nanded.

PREFACE

I

This book on AYUSH in Public Health as presented in two Volumes originates in the understanding of Anthropology in Medicine as a topic under the curriculum of Applied Anthropology at the Masters programme in Anthropology at Sagar University.

The voyages of travellers like Christopher Columbus, Vasco-de-Gama, Marco Polo and others first documented the physical and cultural habits of the people. With the classical field work tradition of Anthropology among the people on islands, or isolated in the forests, valleys and hills, usually referred to as primitives; documentation of queer customs triggered interpretation about the evolution and diffusion of human institutions. If Man was biologically evolved, so would be the institutions of Man. Functionalist theories developed from the observations about Man-Man, Man-Environment and Man-Supernatural relationships providing a unique identity to each Culture. Study of health attitudes, practices developed such sub-disciplines like Ethno-medicine, Ethno-botany or Ethno-biology. Medical Anthropology encompasses all of these indigenous knowledge systems and the implications of modern bio-medicine about health and disease patterns.

In the old world civilizations, more particularly the Asian civilizations, great textual traditions, like Ayurveda, Yoga, Chinese, Unani etc. were developed by the reflective urban elite intellectuals by studying the clinical evidence of their own experiences and of the indigenous healers about the traditional healing practices.

Due to invasions and colonial rule, different systems of medicine proliferated in India. The textual great traditions in healing were available in the referral urban centres. However, the lay people in villages continued and still continue, with their indigenous healing practices for common ailments. Anthropologists prefer to document these as ethno-medicine which do not reach the health bureaucracies, who make policies about health care and implement them. The success of modern bio-medicine in controlling epidemics of communicable diseases has oriented the public sector health care to allopathic system. Ayurved or Unani colleges were established in the princely States of India, not so much in the directly ruled British Presidencies.

The planning process in pre-Independent India about the vision of health care, ideas about Naturopathy by leaders like Mahatma Gandhi, have culminated in the establishment of National ISM&H policy. Parallel systems of health care in some states have now reached the end point of establishment of AYUSH Ministry at Delhi in November 2014.

However, the dynamics of interaction between the Public Sector, Private Sector and People's Sector is not yet being interpreted through research documentation. While the modern pharmaceutical drugs developed through the 'scientific process' of animal trials and clinical trials, they are withdrawn from the market after few years or get banned. The allegations about the efficacy of traditional drugs used by people since long are mounted again and again, due to lack of documentation and epidemiological research.

The present book in two volumes therefore is an attempt from the standpoint of Medical Anthropology to document the practices of common people and the traditional healers, in taking care of the common ailments by themselves. In the second volume, an attempt is made to acquaint the AYUSH practitioners and academics about epidemiological research methods, applicable to AYUSH public health issues. Some research case studies are presented as examples.

Classical Anthropology as holistic study of Man in totality is people-centric, since the central aim is to understand the life as people live it (Culture) through their eyes, through their spectacles. However, since, the patterns of governance in a democratic set-up has changed under the garb of welfare, development and technology, the MACRO is overshadowing the MICRO, the ETIC is controlling the EMIC. As a consequence, anthropological concept of wholeness has to incorporate the different stakeholder perceptions about health and disease, in a broad framework of inter-sectoral co-ordination, provided by Alma Ata declaration of Health For All (HFA), by practicing the Primary Health Care approach, thereby giving the rightful place to traditional medical systems.

The books are meant to provide a pathway for AYUSH epidemiological research in order to provide scientific base to the mood of the humanity to move from Illness to Wellness.

The first volume of this book 'AYUSH in Public Health' has documented the household practices of AYUSH mainly in the four States of India, viz. Himachal Pradesh, Madhya Pradesh, Chhattisgarh and Maharashtra. Similar studies in Rajasthan and 18 other States in India have also been referred which validate the little traditions (local health traditions) with the classical great traditions. The annexures to Volume I detail out the home remedies practiced by people in their homes as also the prescriptions given by local indigenous healers. This brings out clearly the organic, historical link between the little traditions (local health traditions) and great textual tradition.

II

The Department of Indian Systems of Medicine and Homoeopathy (ISM&H) established in March 1995, renamed as Department of AYUSH in November 2003 has been upgraded as an autonomous Ministry of AYUSH in November 2014 under the Ministry of Health and Family Welfare, Government of India. A distinct National AYUSH Mission (NAM) has been launched in September 2014 for the implementation of Strategic Plan of AYUSH mainly in the areas of AYUSH Services by up-gradation of hospitals, dispensaries and co-location at PHC/CHC/DHC, up-gradation of educational institutions, pharmacies and drug testing laboratories.

The mission of AYUSH Ministry has been set-up to mainstream AYUSH at all levels in the Health Care System. The document provides implementation strategies by way of administrative and financial logistics, which fall in the area of bureaucracy.

There has been a reference to Public Health initiatives by way of preparing:

(i) Training material for AYUSH/Allopathic doctors in public health.

(ii) Training of AYUSH/Allopathic doctors in delivery of AYUSH interventions in public health.
(iii) Delivery of AYUSH public health interventions in one or more community blocks for developing AYUSH public health model.
(iv) AYUSH schemes for adolescent girls, women of reproductive age group and geriatric care.
(v) Life Style disorders
(vi) Nutrition and Anemia
(vii) IEC materials in AYUSH

The proposals to be supported would be in the areas of :

(a) Mother-Child Care
(b) Nutrition
(c) Anemia
(d) Epidemiological studies
(e) Training of AYSUH practitioners and paramedics.

Reference has also been made to AYUSH Gram, School Health Programme and the involvement of Panchayati Raj institutions. Proposals are to be focused on bridging the gaps of public health care with AYUSH approach.

Co-laterally, there have been recommendations of the AYUSH Steering Committee for 12th Plan.

Earlier AYUSH was mentioned in the National Health Policy, 1983 and 2002, while a distinct National ISM&H Policy 2002 was also approved. A concerted effort was launched to mainstream AYUSH in Health Care under National Rural Health Mission (NRHM) by way of encouraging co-location of AYUSH facilities with the Primary Health Centre model upwards to district level. An integrated National Health Policy is on the anvil.

The Maharashtra Association of Anthropological Sciences, (MAAS) Pune was granted a project : "Mainstreaming of AYUSH under NRHM", as a proposal under the Central Sector Scheme on Public Health Initiative, in February 2008.Following the presentation of the report of this study project in the four States of Himachal Pradesh, Madhya Pradesh, Chhattisgarh and Maharashtra, a "Centre for AYUSH in Public Health" was granted under the "Central Sector Scheme for Grant-in-aid for Promotion of AYUSH Intervention in Public Health Initiatives" to evolve into a Centre of Excellence, starting as COE (Part) in May 2010, in the States of Himachal Pradesh, Chhattisgarh and Maharashtra.

The biggest challenge for the start-up of the Centre was to develop the vision of AYUSH personnel in administration, Medical Officers in AYUSH Health Centres and AYUSH Medical Institutions, about the role of AYUSH in Public Health, apart from its strength in treatment of afflictions. The need for epidemiology and research training in public health was to be ignited in the AYUSH sector, since AYUSH research was limited to only drug research linked with diseases, not health.

Volume II of the book 'AYUSH in Public Health' has been developed as a Handbook to provide guidelines for undertaking epidemiological training and research in AYUSH Public Health related issues. The handbook essentially documents the training activities undertaken in the three States of Himachal Pradesh, Chhattisgarh and Maharashtra. Some pilot projects undertaken in AYUSH in Public Health issues have also been reported as illustrative case studies. The research formats and training material as also some IEC examples have been included as annexures. The annexures are meant to provide the tools and techniques of public health research in the Do-it-Yourself mode. The road map of replicating such Centre has also been provided as an example.

Unfortunately due to funding crunch, probably as a result of completion of 11th Plan, project development workshops for AYUSH doctors in AYUSH health services and AYUSH medical institutions could not be organized to develop concrete public health research proposals, for submission to AYUSH Ministry, for independent funding to respective research scientists and institutions.

At the same time, it is satisfying that the recommendations by the Centre about AYUSH in Public Health were accepted by the AYUSH Steering Committee for 12th Plan.

The documents generated in the Government sector such as National AYUSH Mission or Strategic Plan do not project Public Health as a priority area in Health Care. They give priority to drug supply and standardization, up-gradation of hospitals and medical education. The High level Expert Group Report on Universal Health Coverage for India Commissioned by the Planning Commission has discussed social determinants of health, community participation, gender issues etc., but there is no focus on AYUSH. AYUSH personnel continue to be numerical manpower to be utilized for disease control and treatment in the PHC system and national health programmes.

However, the utilization of AYUSH at the household level by way of traditional health attitudes and practices regarding treatment of common ailments, maternal and child care and about *Dincharya* and *Ritucharya* validated in the classical texts, being part of culture, calls for AYUSH becoming the mainstream of Public Health. These are not statistically documented and get brushed aside as claims by the health and finance bureaucracies.

Concept of *Prakriti* although accepted now by proponents of individual designer medicine does not get translated to document and analyze public health from AYUSH perspective. It becomes therefore necessary to use the science of Epidemiology to analyze the role of AYUSH in Public Health.

AYUSH systems in India are not a part of PHC/CHC model of health care. Where AYUSH personnel work in PHC, they work in a subordinate position coupled with deficiency in supplies of AYUSH medicine. In the States, where AYUSH health centres are established, they run as parallel institutions offering treatment in the OPD with AYUSH drug. They have no role to play in preventive and promotive care, since they have no networking with sub-centres or the paramedics like ANM, ASHA, Anganwadi workers etc. who actual provide services at the doorstep in the village homes. The traditional herbalist (Vaidu, Baiga, Gunia etc.) who possess indigenous knowledge about herbal medicine, and the TBA (*Dai*) are not co-opted in the formal health care systems and may be shunned as quacks. The concept of institutional delivery works against the use of *Dai* services provided through ages. The Ayurvedic hospitals even at the district level do not have maternity wards.

The AYUSH manpower is considered numerically as health care manpower for contributing to national health programmes without getting any formal credit for it. It becomes therefore imperative that unless AYUSH education, training and research is oriented to Public Health and Epidemiology, AYUSH will continue to be subordinate partners in health care.

We hope, this handbook will provide leads to participate in Public Health issues, using AYUSH strengths presented in the epidemiological format.

III

The beginnings were made when Armed Forces Medical College (AFMC), Pune sought my services to understand the role of social sciences in community health, to the Army Medical Corps (AMC) officers in their postgraduate training in Advanced Preventive Medicine, in the year 1963. I was recommended by a classical anthropologist, Prof. Irawati Karve to undertake the task which continued for three decades. The initiatives of the AFMC were followed by the civil B. J. Medical College, Pune under the leadership of Prof. N. S. Deodhar, Chairman of the Department of Preventive and Social Medicine. In both the institutions, formal appointments as visiting faculty were made respectively by the Defence Ministry and the Government of Maharashtra.

Formal breakthrough about the study of Indian Systems of Medicine (now AYUSH) in Medical Anthropology began with the participation of Prof. Charles Leslie, Prof. A. L. Basham, and Pandit Shiv Sharma at the International Symposium on Medical Anthropology at the Department of Anthropology, University of Pune during 19-21 December, 1978. Prof. H. K. Bhat and Prof. P. C. Joshi who have established Society for Indian Medical Anthropology and who organised a conference in my honour at Mysore in 2007, were two of the few Indian delegates who participated at the Symposium. Prof. Basham organised the first International Conference on Traditional Asian Medicine (ICTAM) at Canberra during September 1979 followed by the establishment of International Association for the Study of Traditional Asian Medicine (IASTAM). IASTAM-India was soon established formally at a meeting at the University of Pune on 27 April, 1980 with Pandit Shiv Sharma as the first President and Prof. R. K. Mutatkar as the first General Secretary.

All these events under the banner of Medical Anthropology, coupled with attempts by Shri Darshan Shankar who established Foundation for Revitalisation of Local Health Traditions (FRLHT) at Banglore, prompted formation of a working group on AYUSH in Public Health under the Chairmanship of Prof. R.K. Mutatkar, to assist the Steering Committee on AYUSH at the XIth Five Year Plan by the Planning Commission. For the first time AYUSH in Public Health became a national agenda.

The two volumes of this book on AYUSH in Public health thus represent the potential strength of Medical Anthropology towards framing and implementation of people centric National Health Policy. We hope, AYUSH would be an active partner in formulating the Mainstream of Health as conceived by the National Rural Health Mission (NRHM). The unified National Health Policy is expected to promote the proven strengths of AYUSH in national health care system.

IV

We have been fortunate in getting the proactive support from the Department of AYUSH, Government of India, towards administering the two projects. We have also been fortunate in getting full cooperation from the respective State Governments. As a policy issue, it was decided to undertake various activities in collaboration with the State Governments, to ensure sustainability of the programme. This also helped to organise project activities economically, since, the subsidized Government and university facilities could be used by the Centre.

In Himachal Pradesh, The Hon. Minister of Health and Ayurved, the OSD in charge of projects, District Ayurved officers and Superintendents of District AYUSH Hospitals, besides the medical officers and paramedical staff at the Ayurvedic Health Centres, need to be specially thanked for their cooperation and affection.

In Chhattisgarh, the Director and OSD of the Department of AYUSH, State Health Resource Centre, Department of Anthropology, Pandit Ravishankar Shukla University, Raipur, and State Medicinal Plant Board, deserve heart-full gratitude. The faculty of Ayurved Medical Colleges, district AYUSH officers, Medical Officers and Paramedical staff including Mitanin, several doctors in charge of Ayurved gram, from all parts of Chhattisgarh, participated in the meetings and provided valuable suggestions.

In Maharashtra, the Director of AYUSH (Medical Education), and Asst. Director, Pune region, Principals and faculty of AYUSH Medical Colleges, and AYUSH doctors in the PHC set-up in Pune district, readily volunteered to initiate the activities. District Health Officers, Health Services Department, need special mention for involving the AYUSH Medical Officers in situation analysis of PHC system. School of Health Sciences, University of Pune was the first to host the vision meeting for AYUSH practitioners and faculty under the Chairmanship of the Dean of Ayurved Faculty.

The members of the Steering and Advisory Committee of the Centre who are very senior scholars drawn across the country took time to deliberate and offer concrete suggestions about the road map that the Centre should follow in mainstreaming AYUSH in National Health Care.

We are confident that this first Centre of AYUSH in Public Health in India will be able to provide leads and insights to other such Centres which need to be established in the National AYUSH Institutes. It would be desirable to establish an independent National Institute of AUYSH in Public Health on lines of National Institute of Epidemiology (ICMR) at Chennai.

Prof. R. K. Mutatkar
Hon. Director,
Centre: AYUSH in Public Health
Maharashtra Association of Anthropological
Sciences (MAAS), Pune

ACKNOWLEDGEMENTS

We are grateful to the initiative taken by Smt. Aneeta Das, Secretary and Sri Shiv Basant, Joint Secretary, Department of AYUSH, Government of India in offering the Mainstreaming study project (volume-I) and deciding the States where the study was to be conducted. Recommended by Sri Shiv Basant, the State Governments of Himachal Pradesh, Madhya Pradesh, Chhattisgarh and Maharashtra helped to select a district for study in the respective States and directed the district AYUSH authorities to accord full co-operation. We were motivated and encouraged by the remark from State officials, "You are doing our work."

The field studies were actually conducted in the two States by the research assistants drawn from the Departments of Anthropology of Dr. Harisingh Gour Vishwavidyalaya, Sagar (M.P.) and Pandit Ravishankar Shukla University, Raipur. Studies in Himachal Pradesh and Maharashtra were undertaken respectively by the research assistants selected by Dr. Rakesh Pandit representing Department of Ayurved, Himachal Pradesh Government, and at the Maharashtra Association of Anthropological Sciences.

Special mention has to be made of the support given by the (Late) Dr. R.S. Arole, Padmabhushan, founder of Jamkhed model of community health, who agreed to the request by Smt. Aneeta Das to be a co-investigator of the Project. He presided over all the meetings held at Pune and graced the meetings at Delhi and Shimla.

Special thanks are due to Dr. Rakesh Pandit of the Department of Ayurved, Himachal Pradesh and Dr. G.S. Badesha, Director of AYUSH, Chhattisgarh, for their personal help at all stages of the investigation.

I personally visited all field sites atleast three times for data collection monitoring, meeting the Government officials in respective States and for presentation of draft reports of each State. The individual State reports have been published in Hindi.

At the national level, Sri Shiv Basant Jt. Secretary, AYUSH had desired the studies in four States conducted by MAAS, a study in Rajasthan by SEDEM and studies in 18 States by NHSRC to be undertaken with a common protocol. In this respect, meetings were held with Dr. Ritu Priya and Dr. Shweta from NHSRC and Dr. Arun Srivastava and Dr. Suhasini from SEDEM at NHSRC, Delhi. I could be present at the orientation of the team leaders for NHSRC from 18 States, held at the School of Oriental Medicine—The Global Open University, Delhi under the leadership of Dr. S.N. Pandey. The publication of SEDEM and NHSRC reports in English and MAAS reports in Hindi, has helped to edit this book in the framework of Medical Anthropology.

We gratefully acknowledge the people of different villages in four States who participated in the research exercise by volunteering to provide information to our research assistants on their practices, opinions and recommendations. We are thankful to the doctors and paramedics who provided their inputs, voiced their concerns and made recommendations which need to be respected, in national interest. We are grateful to all participants at the Stakeholders meetings in different States which provided us the insights about their concerns regarding people centric health care delivery.

Smt. S. Jalaja who followed Smt. Aneeta Das as Secretary was very supportive and encouraged us to do further work by awarding a Centre for AYUSH in Public Health, to develop into a Centre of Excellence. Under Centre for AYUSH in Public Health, our task was to orient the vision of AYUSH medical officers and AYUSH Faculty to undertake epidemiological and public health research about health care and disease control activities. We undertook training sessions about research methods at national and state level and tried some pilot projects in three states as intervention research exercises. We have been helped at national and state levels by the following persons:

We are grateful to:

Department of AYUSH, Government of India

Smt. Aneeta Das, Smt. S. Jalaja, Secretary; Sri Shiv Basant, Joint Secretary; Sri Balaprasad, Sri Premkumar Jha, Sri Rajkumar, Director; Dr. Dinesh Katoch, Dr. Manoj Nesari, Joint Advisor; Dr. Ghose Mondal, Research Officer.

NHSRC

Dr. Sunderraman, Executive Director; Dr. Ritu Priya, Advisor; Dr. Shweta, Consultant.

SEDEM

Dr. Arun Srivastav, Dr. Suhasini.

Steering and Advisory Committee: Centre for AYUSH in Public Health, MAAS.

(Late) Dr. R.S. Arole, Chairman; Sri Darshan Shankar (FRLHT); Dr. Ravi Narayan (SOCHARA); Dr. M. D. Gupte (NIE); Dr. D. C. Katoch & Dr. Manoj Nesari (AYUSH Ministry); (Late) Vd. Vilas Nanal; Father Sebastian (CHAI); Dr. Rakesh Pandit (H.P.); Dr. P. P. Doke & Dr. Sarita Gaikwad (Government of Maharashtra) ; Dr. N. S. Bhatt (IASTAM); and Dr. Babu Joseph (NIN, AYUSH Ministry).

1. **Training of AYUSH MOs & Faculty:** Dr. K. R. Kohli, Director (Maharashtra); Dr. G. S. Badesha, Director (Chhattisgarh); Dr. Rakesh Pandit (OSD Himachal Pradesh); Dr. M. D. Gupte; Dr. Sanjay Mehendale; Dr. Manoj Murhekar (NIE Chennai); Dr. Asha Pratinidhi ; Dr. P. P. Doke (Director, SHRC); Dr. Ramesh Paranjpe (Director NARI); Dr. Radhika Brhame (NARI); Dr. V. K. Mehta (Shimla), Dr. Soni Kapil (Shimla), Dr. Anita Sharma (Una); Dr. Harjindar Singh (Una); Dr. Rita Bherwal (Una); Dr. Arun Dabake, (V. C. Ayurved & Health University, Raipur); Prof. R. K. Ram (PSM); J. N. Medical College, Raipur; Dr. S.L. Gupta, Consultant, SHRC, Raipur; Dr Saurabh Jain, SHRC, Raipur.

Himachal Pradesh

Dr. Rajeev Bindal, Hon. Minister of Health and Ayurved; Dr. Rakesh Pandit, OSD, Ayurved ; Dr. Jagirsingh Pathania, Dr. Avinash Gupta, DAO, Hamirpur and Una; Dr. Hemraj Sharma,

Research Co-ordinator, Dr. B. D. Soni, Dr. Daljitsingh Banyal and Dr. Subhash Chandla, Medical Officer.

Madhya Pradesh

Sri Mukesh Varshney, Commissioner AYUSH; Dr. Anup Khare, DAO, Sagar; Prof. A. N. Sharma, Professor of Anthropology, Dr. Harisingh Gaur Vishwavidyalaya, Sagar.

Chhattisgarh

Dr. G. S. Badesha, Director, AYUSH; Dr. Vijay Sahu, OSD; Dr. M. L. Tekchandani, Dr. Pradeep Shukla, DAO, Bilaspur; Dr. Nilesh Jain, Co-ordinator, AYUSH, SHRC, Prof. Mitashree Mitra, Professor of Anthropology, Pt. Ravishankar Shukla University, Raipur, Dr. Laknesh Sharma, Dr. S. P. Singh, Dr. Pritam Sharma, Medical Officers, Ayurved; Dr. Sameer Tiwari, AMO Ayurved Gram Nimdha; Dr. R. N. Pati, UNDP, Raipur, Dr. Devangan, AMO, Korba, and Dr. Sushila Banjare, AMO, Hirri.

Maharashtra

Dr. K. R. Kohli, Director, AYUSH (Medical Education); Dr. Sarita Gaikwad, Asst. Director; Dr. P.P. Doke, Director SHRC ; Dr. R.S. Arole, Padmabhushan, Jamkhed Shri G. S. Pandit, Dr. Shailesh Dalvi, Dr. Sanjay Dakhore MAAS; Dr. Kalpana Mutatkar, Consultant, MAAS; Dr. Robin Tribhuvan, Medical anthropologist, Nagesh Bangare, Tribal Vaidu, practitioner and trainer; Dr. V. V. Doiphode, Chairman Rashtriya Arogya Mandal; Dr. Tanuja Nesari, Principal, Tilak Ayurved College; Dr. Saroj Patil, Dr. Mihir Hajarnavis, Dr. Manoj Gaikwad, Dr. Mohan Joshi, Dr. Swati Gaikwad, Dr. Vinay Dixit, Dr. Indira Ujagare, Dr. A. M. Sangoram Dr. Sujata Kadam, Tilak Ayurved College; Dr. Farah Sikalgar & Dr. Nasrin Shaikh, Unani Collage, Pune; Dr. Satish Dumbre, Principal, Ashtang Ayurved Mahavidyalay and Dean, Ayurved, MUHS, Nashik.

Dr. Robin Tribhuvan, medical anthropologist working as Senior Research officer at the Tribal Research and Training Institute of the Government of Maharashtra took special leave and visited all field sites to monitor the field research exercise and submitted reports immediately. His interviews with the *Dais* (TBA) in three States about fetal growth have been exemplary. Dr. Shailesh Dalvi (MAAS), an ayurvedic physician by training, collected and analyzed the data from tribal centres in Maharashtra. Administrative support for computer processing of data and text, as also accounting was provided by MAAS.

Field Investigation Teams

- **Himachal Pradesh:** Smt. Neeta Sharma, Smt. Parvin Kumari, Subhash Chand, Sunil Kumar.
- **Madhya Pradesh:** Smt. Rachana Thakur, Arjunsingh Thakur, Ashishkumar Yadav, Sandeepprasad Daksha.
- **Chhattisgarh:** Smt. Anita Minj, Smt. Shradha Sahu, Rajeshkumar Dubey, Ajay Sahu.
- **Maharahstra:** Umesh, Patil, Nagesh, Pavra, Vasave, Vyavhare, Khandare, Durge, Telore (Nine tribal centres).

MAAS

Write up: Drafts of data sets were made by respective field teams. Research Coordinators, Raghavendra Madhu, Rajesh Dubey and Prachi Kumar systematized and translated the qualitative data sets in English. Programme Co-ordinator, Centre for AYUSH in Public Health, Dr. Devendra Sonawne, Dr. Sarika Kadam, systematized home remedies according to disease condition as per principles of Ayurved and correlated the local names with Botanical terms. Her technical support has been exemplary. Dr. Sucheta Marne undertook analysis of field data.

Computer processing: Smt. Aarti Pardeshi, Smt. Sharvari Nisal, Smt. Swati Dandare, Nandu Dighe (DTP and publication of Hindi reports). Special mention has to be made about the dedication of Smt. Sharvari Nisal about the maintenance of academic and administrative records and typing of letters and reports, and to make the soft and hard copies available on demand, at short notice.

Accounts: Smt. Anisha Dhongade, Shri J. J. Dange, Vinayak Amle.

CONTENTS

LIST OF ABBREVIATIONS AND ACRONYMS

AFMC	=	Armed Forces Medical College
AHC	=	Ayurvedic Health Centre
ANC	=	Anti Natal Care
ANM	=	Auxiliary Nurse Midwife
ASHA	=	Accredited Social Health Activist
ASU	=	Ayurved, Siddha, Unani
AUK	=	Adivasi Utthan Karyakram
AWW	=	Anganwadi Worker
AYUSH	=	Ayurveda, Yoga and Naturopathy, Unani, Siddha and Homoeopathy
BCC	=	Behavioural Change Communication
BPL	=	Below Poverty Line
CBO	=	Community Based Organization
CCIM	=	Central Council of Indian Medicine
CCRAS	=	Central Council for Research in Ayurveda and Siddha
CCRAS	=	Central Council for Research in Ayurvedic Sciences
CCRUM	=	Central Council for Research in Unani Medicine
CCRUS	=	Central Council for Research in Unani Siddha
CHC	=	Community Health Centre
CRHP	=	Comprehensive Rural Health Project, Jamkhed
FPAI	=	Family Planning Association of India
FRCH	=	Foundation for Research in Community Health
FRLHT	=	Foundation for Revitalisation of Local Health Traditions
GMLF	=	Gandhi Memorial Leprosy Foundation
GoI	=	Government of India
Govt.	=	Government
GP	=	General Practice
HMIS	=	Health Management Information System
IASTAM	=	International Association for the Study of Traditional Asian Medicine
IASTAM-India		International Association for the Study of Traditional Asian Medicine-India chapter

ICDS	=	Integrated Child Development Services
ICMR	=	Indian Council of Medical Research
ICTAM	=	International Congress on Traditional Asian Medicine
IEC	=	Information, Education and Communication
INCAA	=	Indian National Confederation and Academy of Anthropologists
IPHS	=	Indian Public Health Standards
ISM	=	Indian Systems of Medicine
ISM&H	=	Indian Systems of Medicine and Homoeopathy
JNU	=	Jawaharlal Nehru University
LHT	=	Local Health Traditions
LSHTM	=	London School of Hygiene & Trophical Medicine
MAAS	=	Maharashtra Association of Anthropological Sciences
MCH	=	Mother and Child Health
MO	=	Medical Officer
MoHFW	=	Ministry of Health and Family Welfare
MPW	=	Multipurpose worker
NCAER	=	National Council of Applied Economic Research
NFHS	=	National Family Health Survey
NGO	=	Non-Governmental Organization
NHSRC	=	National Health Systems Resource Centre
NRHM	=	National Rural Health Mission
NSSO	=	National Sample Survey Organization
OPD	=	Out Patient Department
PHC	=	Primary Health Centre
PNC	=	Post-Natal Care
PRI	=	Panchayati Raj Institutions
RCH	=	Reproductive and Child Health
RH	=	Rural Hospital
SC	=	Sub Centre
SEDEM	=	Society for Economic Development and Environmental Management
SHG	=	Self-Help Group
SHRC	=	State Health Resource Centre
SIMA	=	Society for Indian Medical Anthropology
ST	=	Scheduled Tribes
TBA	=	Traditional Birth Attendant
TM	=	Traditional Medicine
UG	=	Undergraduate
VHSC	=	Village Health and Sanitation Committee
WHO	=	World Health Organization

1
PROLOGUE
National Perspective

Health from the social science perspective refers to the total fitness of an individual which would ensure performance of social roles to optimum efficiency. All societies equip their members through the processes of socialization and enculturation to play useful roles commensurate with their statuses. Society also provides institutional mechanism to look after the sick with a view to minimize the period and extent of disability and maximize the quantum of recovery in shortest possible period.

Health is an aspect of culture, that is, way of life of a group or a community equivalent to economic, political, social and religious aspects of life. All these aspects are interrelated as structural and functional parts of the culture which is an integrated whole. Health aspects could be classified into 'soft core of health culture' or visible, material aspects such as treatment with medicine. The 'hard core of health culture' is represented by ideas about prevention and promotion of health and ideas about causation of illness which could be in the areas of faith and belief. Cause-effect relationship about health and illness could, therefore, fall in the areas of cultural belief system. The treatment therapies are in the realm of soft aspects or material aspects of culture. The plural treatment therapies may be herbal or animal, marine and mineral elements, or synthetic drugs in modern medicine, which are adopted by clinical experience. Magico-religious procedures are also followed in health and illness, sometimes in conjunction with drug therapy. Whatever may be the perception of causes of ill health, people accept treatment which provides affordable remedy as fast as possible. Use of mobile phones does not necessarily mean acceptance of the scientific aspects of communication technology or does not help to imbibe scientific temper. There is no vacuum of perceived knowledge or practices in matters of health and medicine in any society. Every citizen shares the attitudes and information about health and disease, and about the medicinal and nutritional values of food, and about healthy or unhealthy environment, with the members of the social group. There is a legend about Birbal telling Akbar that the Hakim was the largest knowledge group in the Empire. When asked to prove the claim, Emperor was advised to feign illness. Every citizen who called on to inquire Akbar's health offered a piece of advice about treatment, care about life style, food etc. to regain and maintain good health. Every citizen proved to be a Hakim.

Indigenous systems of medicine as are practiced in the folk or tribal society and practiced as home remedies in the mainstream society are linked with the textual medicine as given in the classical texts like—Charak, Sushrut, Vagbhat and such similar Unani or Siddha texts.

In Anthropology, Robert Redfield tried to understand the civilizations as continuing interaction between the Little traditions as practiced by lay people and Great tradition enshrined in the scriptures or mythologies. Great tradition refers to the literate tradition of a civilization which is developed and maintained by the reflective elite and intellectual class of the society. Little tradition refers to the culture and customs followed by the peasant society, which is linked to great tradition as a referral value.

A case in point are the *Gita, Ramayana* and *Mahabharata* among the Hindu, the *Bible* among the Christians, the *Quran* among the Muslims and such other scriptures among other religious groups such as the Jains, Buddhists and Sikhs. There have been any number of commentaries on *Gita* over the centuries including those by personalities like Shankaracharya, Dnyaneshwar (Gynaneshwar), Tilak, Gandhi, Vinoba and many others linking philosophical values to issues in practical life, thus linking the little and great traditions. *Gita* continues to be interpreted in small village temples as well as in five star hotels. Leprosy scientific meetings of Christian organizations invariably open with passages from *Bible* linking with dedicated work in leprosy healing and control. Thus, Bible messages are discussed for motivation in work.

The concepts of Little tradition and Great tradition could be used to analyze the interaction and validation of the health practices followed by the people as home remedies and as given in the classical texts. Currently, the term "local health traditions" is being widely used for home remedies in public documents. The term has gained currency due to efforts of Foundation for Research in Local Health Traditions (FRLHT), Bangalore, initiated by Shri Darshan Shankar whose team started work on these issues at the Academy of Development Science in the tribal belt around Kashele, Tahsil Karjat, District Raigad, Maharashtra, not very far from the metropolis of Mumbai. However, the concepts of Little tradition and Great tradition enunciated by an anthropologist Robert Redfield, are based on analytical studies of great civilizations like the Indian and Chinese, and his field studies undertaken in Mexico.

The studies referred in the book focus mainly on the home remedies and indigenous healers and para-professionals in the rural areas in Himachal Pradesh, Madhya Pradesh, Chhattisgarh and Maharashtra by The Maharashtra Association of Anthropological Sciences (MAAS), Pune, highlighting the little traditions or local health traditions in the respective States. The study also documented health systems or health care delivery in the public sector. A similar study was undertaken in Rajasthan by Society for Economic Development and Environmental Management (SEDEM), New Delhi. National Health Systems Resource Centre (NHSRC) undertook studies in 18 States of India, not covered by MAAS and SEDEM, which also brought out peoples' knowledge and practices about home remedies. The studies undertaken by MAAS have been more qualitative in nature following the anthropological methods of field investigations covering the whole universe of the selected villages. The Rajasthan and NHSRC studies have been more quantitative and also cover the providers' perspectives and health care delivery systems in the public and private domain.

Both Rajasthan study by SEDEM and NHSRC studies in 18 States are focused on Health Systems Research in the context of NRHM's objective of bringing in co-location of different systems of medicine. However, since the studies were designed to understand the position of AYUSH with the ideal objective of mainstreaming AYUSH in Health Care Delivery, recommendations are weighted in favour of capacity building of paramedics and of the doctors, dealing with health issues of women, children and elderly about AYUSH. NHSRC studies have analyzed the statistics in regard to use of home remedies by community in common ailments, use of folk healers, TBA use during pregnancy, delivery and lactation and about the knowledge of medicinal plants and medicinal properties of food items. All these home remedies, medicinal plants and food items with medicinal properties, perceived by the households, have been validated using documented codified knowledge of AYUSH systems. "Here 'validation' was taken as verifying the content of formal providers' prescriptions and people's knowledge of medicinal plants and foods, as well as home remedies in light of AYUSH epistemology and documented codified knowledge" (NSHRC: 2010: 160-171). This research finding is of great value to counter the argument, to treat AYSUH as unscientific or non-rational, unless otherwise proved by laboratory based clinical trials.

The publications by CCRAS and CCRUS about "An Appraisal of Tribal Folk Medicine (1999)", "Handbook of Domestic Medicine and Common Ayurvedic Remedies"(2005) and "Handbook of Common Remedies in Unani System of Medicine" (2003) are useful references. A paper by Vaidya Antarkar on "The use of scientifically validated herbs and plants in primary health care"(ICMR: 1981: 79-86) is another good resource.

However, both SEDEM and NHSRC studies have not given the qualitative details of home remedies. MAAS studies in four States identified by the AYUSH Department have focused on the use of AYUSH by the people and not so much on the use of AYUSH Health Care Delivery. The ethnographic method using the tools of non-formal interviews, observation, key informant interviews have documented the spontaneous narrations about the use of herbs, their combinations in common ailments and in Mother and Child Health Care etc. The names of ailments, plants, processing of herbs to be used as medicine etc. are given in detail. One ANM in Himachal Pradesh exclaimed that her kitchen was her home dispensary. If she did not get relief there, she would use her ANM medicine. The Minister of Health and Ayurved in Himachal Pradesh, himself an Ayurvedic physician, sought our recommendation to mainstream home remedies in the formal health care delivery system. MAAS did not probe in depth about the collocation aspects which did not appear to be visible. Even co-located AYUSH systems did not engage themselves in cross-referencing, although located in the adjacent rooms in a big multi-storeyed Regional AYUSH hospital of the Government.

The three institutions were advised by the Secretary and Joint Secretary, AYUSH Department, Government of India to follow a similar protocol for study. As reported by SEDEM in its Rajasthan report, "Subsequently, the institution was requested to coordinate with NHSRC (Dr. Ritu Priya) and Dr. R.K. Mutatkar to develop a joint research plan to document utilization pattern of home remedies, LHT, and the manner in which State Governments are integrating Allopathic and AYUSH systems. This modified our original proposal" (SEDEM: 2010: 1). Initially there was close communication and meetings among the three institutions to develop and standardize the tools of data collection. However, MAAS with the help of anthropology departments focused on qualitative studies using the study tools as guides rather than for collection of statistical data. The strength of NHSRC studies lies in the textual validation of home remedies and the prescriptions of AYUSH doctors. All the studies in 23 States bring out the fact of wide utilization of AYUSH home remedies and AYUSH services by the people for primary health care.

Ironically, the Department of AYUSH, Government of India is asked to defend on the point of utilization of AYUSH by the people, for seeking budgetary allocation from the Finance and Planning Departments. Since AYUSH medicines are used as home remedies on a large scale as little traditions and are also made by the Vaidyas and Hakims at home based clinics, as also by traditional herbalists or *dais*, it is not possible to get the authentic statistical data about utilization. Since, the allopathic medicines are essentially manufactured in licensed pharmacies and also sold in licensed shops, the purchase of medicines by the people is documented at various stages from production to sale by way of taxes collected by the government.

NHSRC Report has discussed this issue in detail: "The Department of AYUSH does not report utilization data. The NSSO and National Council of Applied Economic Research (NCAER) health surveys provide some of the national level data on utilization of health services. However, the recent rounds of NSSO do not consider AYUSH services separately at all, and home remedies are clubbed with 'no treatment' (NSSO). The NFHS too does not take into consideration the utilization of AYUSH services, since in its categorization of "treatment was sought from a health facility or provider" it "excludes pharmacy, shop, and traditional practitioner" (NFHS). The NFHS does have some data on home and herbal remedies in relation to diarrhoeal disease in children and on general sources of health care in households, but its findings are at marked variance with the large body of literature on health seeking behaviours from research in medical anthropology and international health systems research, since the NFHS-3 finds that only 8 per cent of children with diarrhoeal disease received such remedies."

"The data on general sources of health care does not have a category of public sector AYUSH services, though it does have traditional systems in the private sector and there it finds utilization for 0.2-0.5 per cent ailments. Thus, while clearly there is an exclusion of traditional systems and folk forms of treatment in the national surveys, it needs to be examined whether there is actually no or very limited demand for AYUSH services, home and herbal remedies, or is this a methodological limitation of these surveys? (NHSRC: 2010: 6, 7) Padam Singh, R.J. Yadav and Arvind Pandey in their papers on "Utilization of indigenous systems of medicine and homoeopathy in India" have reported 33 per cent of the 45000 sick persons from 33,666 households from 35 districts preferring AYUSH for common ailments while 18 per cent preferred use in care of serious ailments (*Indian J. Med Res.* 122, August 2005: 137-142).

Actually, eliciting data about utilization at the household level depends upon the method or tool of seeking information. If a question is asked in a schedule or a questionnaire, as to whether Ayurved or Unani or Naturopathy is used by family members the answer could be negative. But if it is asked as to what home remedies have been tried for specific problems like cough, cold or joint pain or during pregnancy etc., the names of herbs and the method of use would be spelt out. The terms for medical systems are given by providers and not by the people. The names of the herbs etc. given by the people are in the domain of little tradition while the terms for the systems are in the domain of great tradition. The same herbs could be used and listed in various medical systems and even listed as home remedies on the internet providing relief for ailments. Lay people do not label them as an Ayurvedic or

Unani product. However, the classical texts discuss the herbs, their processing as single or part of plural drug and relate them to respective theories about body metabolism. It has been observed that the century old shops selling Ayurvedic or Unani medicinal herbs are visited by the people to purchase items over the counter to prepare herbal products for therapy or for promotive health. They identify the shops by location or by the name of the owner and not necessarily by system of medicine. Some of the common spices available in grocery shops are purchased from these medicinal shops if the product is to be used as medicine and not as kitchen spices, particularly in respect of maternal and child health.

In addition to the NHSRC and SEDEM field studies, Smt. Shailaja Chandra, Former Secretary, Department of AYUSH, Government of India, undertook a review of "Status of Indian Medicine and Folk Healing" presented in two parts and has made significant recommendations about operationalising AYUSH systems as mainstream health system.

The exercise of undertaking the studies by MAAS was initiated as a result of Steering Committee report on AYUSH for the Eleventh Five Year Plan and as a result of recommendation of mainstreaming AYUSH under National Rural Health Mission (NRHM).

The ethnographic studies conducted by MAAS in the four States are in line with the tradition of ethnography in anthropological research. With the rise of Medical Anthropology in mid-seventies, field studies of health behaviour and healing practices and the studies of indigenous healers among various ethnic tribal groups and caste Hindu peasant villages have been increasing. Ethno-botany, Ethno-physiology have developed as collateral disciplines of Ethnology and Ethnography.

Several research papers documenting the ethnography of cultural health practices and health services provided by the traditional healers are presented at the seminars and conferences organized by the Departments of Anthropology across the country. Academic organizations like Society for Indian Medical Anthropology (SIMA) and Indian National Confederation and Academy of Anthropologists (INCAA) at their conferences have invariably sessions on traditional medicine. However, the data sets so generated are not taken into account for policy formulation. There is no meaningful dialogue between the policy planners and academics. Actually, the faculty and students as also private clinicians practicing AYUSH, trained formally as per classics of Great Tradition are aware that the Little traditions followed in Indian homes have had an interactive relationship between the two traditions for ages. But this awareness does not get translated into a dialogue with the folk healers, herbalists and *dais* (TBA). Local healers do not get the advantage of up-scaling their indigenous knowledge with great tradition. Professionally trained AYUSH physicians have a lower self esteem if they are identified not different from herbalists. They are seen acclaiming that Ayurved, Unani, Siddha were not herbalist disciplines. They are not willing to accept that the little traditions and great traditions are the two ends of a knowledge continuum which sustains a civilization.

However, the resurgence of national health movement in India, concurrent with the Independence movement, and with the institutionalization of Naturopathy blessed by Mahatma Gandhi, and Yoga as therapeutic and health system getting international accreditation, has opened the avenues for a single National Health Policy in India. Primary Health Care Approach of "Health for All" by WHO, triggered partly by Chinese primacy to Chinese system of medicine made visible by 'barefoot doctor' helped to establish Division of Traditional Medicine at the WHO, Geneva.

This book documenting the knowledge and practice of home remedies as guided by elders and indigenous healers, would provide much needed evidence about the widespread utilization of AYUSH. To repeat again, even at the highest level of budget justification, AYUSH Department is asked to defend budgetary requirement in terms of utilization of AYUSH products and services by the people. People do not brand the little traditions of home practiced and produced therapy or utilization of the services of traditional healers by a system of medicine, such as Ayurved, Unani or Siddha, but identify these as traditional home remedies. The Great tradition brands are intellectual creations of the literati generalized from the evidence based little traditions of the masses. How can these practices be transformed into statistical digits for comparison with allopathic products which are not produced except in a pharmaceutical factory, sold in shops and countable due to taxes levied at various levels?

The maternity practices of lady doctors from all systems of medicine who follow the cultural, traditional practices, when they become mothers themselves, could be measured in statistical terms. To a formal question, some of them could answer that they followed these practices under the social pressure of mother-in-law and affectionate pressure of mother. However, informally they also admit that they and the babies benefited from traditional practices or at worst had no bad side effects. National multi-centric ethnographic studies of plural medical systems with good case studies would provide rich data on the subject.

In this context, the quantitative and qualitative studies in 23 States in India document the massive evidence of use of validated products and practices of AYUSH followed by the people. The need of the people to get the advantage of historically evolved plural systems of medicine in India could be met by instituting an integrated national health system. This would require architectural redesigning of health institutions, medical education and the enhanced and empowered use of community based paramedics in health care. What is being followed by the people in their homes as little traditions of AYUSH has to be mainstreamed by way of formal training of great AYUSH traditions in the medical and paramedical curricula.

The barefoot doctor model of China, the Jamkhed model of Dr. R.S. Arole in Maharashtra which have already created Community Health Volunteers, Health Guides, ANM, Anganwadi workers and now ASHA could develop holistic integrated Indian model of health care, which could connect, upscale and strengthen peoples' indigenous knowledge of health care.

The issues of health and disease at the individual, family and community level revolve around the home based health care, health care services provided by traditional healers, and by professionally trained doctors and experienced para-medics in the private sector, and now, the health care delivery in the public sector by plural medical systems in a parallel mode.

This book discusses these issues with primary data collected by the anthropological-ethnographic tools and techniques in four States by MAAS and supplemented by studies in eighteen States undertaken by NHSRC and one study by SEDEM. The book thus provides an all India perspective of Little traditions duly validated by Great textual tradition which need to be taken into account while formulating and implementing the single holistic National Health Policy, which would offer plural choices to the people with requisite knowledge about the strengths of each system.

In addition, there is discussion about the Health Systems or Health Care Delivery in the public and private sector including about AYUSH medical education. The NHSRC and SEDEM reports have dwelt more on AYUSH Health Systems respectively in 18 States and Rajasthan with relevant statistics collected through quantitative methods.

This book is expected to generate more multi-centric research based on primary data which should prove useful for advocacy to provide AYUSH the prime position in primary health care instead of treating it as a subsidiary or alternate or complementary system.

This book on AYUSH community health in primary health care is an attempt to present an all India utilization, and perspective based on studies undertaken in 23 States by three organizations, in consultation with the Deportment of AYUSH, Government of India, following a common protocol of study. Each of the three studies have its own strength, but put together provide insights useful for policy formulation.

The book is presented in Chapters, and annexures providing the names of home remedies, herbs and their processing at household level as also used by the traditional local herbalists. Introduction discusses anthropological perspectives of health as an aspect of culture and the rise of traditional medicine as formal health care system at the national and international level. It thus provides a pathway for national health policy planning and its implementation ensuring community participation.

Chapter on Study Design provides the objectives of the three studies and the emic approach of MAAS study and etic approaches of NHSRC and SEDEM studies. Put together, the outcome provides a holistic perspective of health care system assessing the mainstreaming of AYUSH under NRHM. Chapter on People's Sector provides home remedy practices by people in 4 States studied by MAAS, practices and concepts of *Dai* about fetal growth, and practices followed by traditional healers about common ailments. The Public Sector in the next chapter provides insights about the government institutions such as PHC, Sub-centre, AYUSH Health Centres. The para-medics like ANM, MPW, AWW, ASHA have very close links with the rural communities, by way of their recruitment and by way of providing direct services in rural homes. Although they are not formal employees in government administrative pattern, they are accountable to the health administration and receive some honorarium from public exchequer. Ideally, these para-professional personnel should functionally be a part of People's Sector, accountable to the people. Chapter on Private Sector provides information about Private doctors or providers of therapy including the Chemist shops which are widely used by people for purchasing drugs over the counter, as suggested by the shop pharmacist.

In each of the four States studied by MAAS, joint meetings of the formal and non-formal health care providers, along with district level and State level health administrators were held to discuss various perspectives. The recommendations from various stakeholders at these meetings or at individual level were encouraged which have been documented.

Epilogue discusses the findings of the studies of 23 States, with recommendations evolved from these studies for realistic health care planning and logistics of implementation under the directions provided by the Constitution about governance. The roles of NGOs, CBOs, SHGs and more importantly of the PRI are discussed to translate the vision and mission into a pathway for better health of the people, utilizing the strengths of plural medical systems available in India.

The book hopes to encourage several multi-centric, national studies making judicious use of both quantitative and qualitative tools of research investigation.

2
INTRODUCTION
Health Culture and AYUSH

I

All living beings through survival instinct maintain equilibrium with the environment for health care. Human beings, however, live more through acquired behaviour than instinctive behaviour. The biological instincts are common to humanity but the acquired response to address the instincts are plural, what is usually referred to as culture. The relationships of Man to Man, Man to Environment and Man to Supernatural have commonalities due to 'Psychic Unity of Mankind', and variations due to historical processes in varied geographical conditions.

There are multitudes of health care practices based on the concepts about body, mind, environment and supernatural world in all human groups. In the old world civilizations of India, China, Greece or Egypt, medical traditions were developed with the concepts of humors such as '*Vata*', '*Pitta*', and '*Kapha*' in Ayurved or '*Yin*' and '*Yang*' in Chinese medicine. The basic framework of Unani Tibb or Graeco-Arab medicine "consists of the four humour theory of Hippocrates, which presupposes the presence in the body of four humours; blood, phlegm, yellow bile, and black bile". Health was expressed in terms of opposite characters such as hot-cold, heavy-light, wet-dry etc. Illness referred to disequilibrium among the humors which needed correction through interventions of therapy in the form of food prescriptions or restrictions, and use of products from the environment having medicinal properties, may be in the form of herbs, minerals or animal products. These in the old world developed great medical traditions which were codified as texts, such as Charak, Sushrut, Vagbhat. This also developed into formal medical education in ancient Universities such as at Nalanda and Takshshila in India as '*Guru-Shishya Parampara*' (Teacher-Student traditional relationship), which continues today, essentially in music and sometimes in therapeutics, also at the doctoral level in academics.

However, access to the scholastic medical knowledge and services in the past, remained limited to the urban literati or as referrals for others. Majority of the tribal people and peasantry used the services of folk healers who had indigenous knowledge generally referred to as local health traditions or little traditions. The masters codified these little or local traditions into the textual great traditions and counselled the students to learn about health practices from everybody including the shepherds who had closer association to the herbs and trees than the peasant cultivators. "The goatherds, shepherds, cowherds and other forest dwellers know the medicinal herbs in the forest by their name and form" (*Charaksamhita* in NHSRC, 2010: 170).

With the development of modern science, knowledge about anatomy, physiology; classification of herbs, minerals, food items and germs, took a new dimension to what is referred as modern medicine or allopathy. With political power and colonial rule, the victors and their knowledge and material culture were identified as superior. Modern medicine got referred to as scientific medicine and other great traditional systems such as Ayurvedic, Chinese or Arabic as non-scientific or at best as ethno-medicine.

Rise of Communist China as a political power and use of the concept of 'barefoot doctor' influenced WHO to include traditional medicine in the 'Alma Ata' declaration about 'Health For All' in 1978, "In China the extensive use of traditional medicine in a modern system of health services has attracted worldwide attention. The system of colleges, research institutes, and other facilities for humoral medicine in India has been created by entrepreneurial practitioners of traditional medicine, and by their patrons in politics, industry, and other modern occupations" (Leslie, 1976: 7).

WHO formally instituted Traditional Medicine Programme at Geneva. The Alma Ata declaration with an objective of total medical coverage for all peoples by the year 2000 has been expressed. To quote "The old debate between advocates of scientific excellence and the champions of minimum effective coverage has been largely resolved by a general consensus that all citizens have a right to health and to medical care of their choice, and that this right should embrace safe maternity, the healthy growth and development of children, maintenance of health in adult life, the protection of individuals and the community from environmental hazards, and the provision of medical care for the sick."

"The debate, however, has taken place mainly between the doctors and the administrators, most of whom think in terms of the technological and organizational assumptions of modern medicine and public health. This background leads many, even of those who are sympathetic to traditional medicine, to think of it as no more than a possibly useful source of manpower to increase the coverage of official health services. Traditional practitioners, many of whom have suffered from official neglect or even persecution, have expressed grave doubts about this relationship" (WHO, 1983: 107).

The relationships between the official and traditional health care services are in the categories of 'monopolistic' (in favour of allopathy), 'tolerant' (of alternative curative medicine, not public health), 'parallel' (as separate systems as in India) and 'integrated' (merged in medical education and jointly practised).

These relationships and attitudes are visible in the Indian scenario. India, however, accepts WHO definition of traditional medicine as including diverse health practices, approaches, knowledge and beliefs incorporating plant, animal, and/or mineral based medicines, spiritual therapies, manual techniques and exercises applied singularly or in combination to maintain well-being, as well as to treat, diagnose or prevent illness (WHO, 2002: 7).

II

Anthropology as a holistic study of Man and His Works, developed as a distinct bio-cultural discipline out of the ethnographic studies of isolated communities, commonly branded as tribal communities. The central concept of culture, that is, way of life which is historically designed encompasses all aspects of life, material and non-material, rational and non-rational. Health as an aspect of culture was not specifically studied since it permeates all practices about food and nutrition, maternity and child rearing, treatment for ill-health and beliefs and faith, which are documented in the respective domains of life. Health as a distinct aspect got research and documentation attention due to institutionalization of health care delivery in the public sector at national and international levels. The control of communicable diseases to arrest epidemics, and sanitation, particularly in urban areas, required governance at various levels. Establishment of WHO and health ministries gave a fillip to scientific research and administration addressing disease control programmes. Health issues and institutionalization got integrated with development issues, focusing rural areas through Community Development Programmes in India.

Anthropological studies of tribal communities followed by village studies did not specifically document health culture as an aspect of community culture. However, the functioning of government health centres as a result of Bhore Committee recommendations, brought in the paramedics directly in contact with the people. The local indigenous healers and *Dais* were providing health care services in a traditional way. Modern medicine made its entry in rural areas through government health care delivery system. This resulted in people having plural access to modern medicine as also folk remedies from the traditional healers in addition to home remedies.

Medical Anthropology as a sub-discipline developed focusing on ethnography of traditional practices and healers, as also on the process of government health care delivery. Anthropology as an academic discipline traditionally studying the micro-level situations with emic perspectives has been producing ethnographic accounts about health care, beliefs and services, under the banner of Medical Anthropology. The post-international congress symposium on Medical Anthropology held at Pune University in December 1978 discussed Medical Pluralism, the proceedings of which were brought out as an international publication of a journal 'Social Science and Medicine' as a special issue edited by Charles Leslie. The International Congress of Anthropological and Ethnological Sciences was held at New Delhi preceding the Medical Anthropology symposium at Pune. The symposium was inaugurated by Dr. C.G. Pandit, First Director, ICMR and was graced by Prof. Charles Leslie, Pandit Shiv Sharma, Prof. A.L. Basham, Prof. Arthur Kleinman and about 50 medical anthropologists from U.S. and Europe. The symposium motivated the formation of an international and later Indian Association for the Study of Traditional Asian Medicine (IASTAM), and Society for Indian Medical Anthropology (SIMA). The conferences of these academic organizations discuss the issue of AYUSH according to their perspectives.

Earlier, Medical Anthropology became a part of Masters Course in Anthropology for the first time in India in 1974 at Pune University. This was facilitated due to Prof. Irawati Karve deputing a lecturer in Social Anthropology, R.K. Mutatkar to engage guest lectures at the Preventive Medicine Department of the Armed Forces Medical College since 1963. The then Prof. Col. B. Mahadevan, Head of the Department who later became the General Commandant of AFMC continued this tradition for three decades. Prof. N.S. Deodhar, Head of the Department of Preventive and Social Medicine, B.J. Medical College, Pune who later became Director, All India Institute of Public Health and Hygiene, Calcutta (now Kolkata) incorporated anthropological aspects of health at the post-graduate curricula in Preventive and Social Medicine. This was immediately followed by Gandhi Memorial Leprosy Foundation, Wardha exposing the field of leprosy to social aspects of leprosy. Thus, leprosy became the first agenda in Medical Anthropology in India, and later at the WHO, Geneva. These social science initiatives in leprosy were blessed by Dr. C.G. Pandit, Padma Bhushan, first Director ICMR, Dr. R.V. Wardekar, Padma Shri, first Director GMLF, Baba Amte, Padma Vibhushan, and Sri Devendra Kumar, Secretary, Gandhi Memorial Fund (Gandhi Smarak Nidhi). Involvement of medical anthropology in community health was initiated by Dr. Banoo Coyaji, Padma Bhushan, who had participated in the Pune symposium on medical anthropology, Dr. N.H. Antia, Padma Shri, and Dr. R.S. Arole, Padma Bhushan which enriched Practicing Medical Anthropology, through inputs in research and training.

Medical anthropology has been defined in various terms such as:

1. Bio-cultural understanding of man and his works in relation to health and medicine.
2. Encompasses the State of medical phenomena as they are influenced by social and cultural features and social and cultural phenomena, as they are illuminated by their medical aspects.

3. Medical anthropologists describe their work relating to (a) research about description and interpretation of bio-cultural interrelationships between human behaviour, health and disease levels, (b) their professional participation in health improvement programmes and programmes about changing health behaviour to promote better health.

Most of the books under the title Medical Anthropology have published papers relating to beliefs and practices of isolated communities or the folk practices of traditional peasant communities. Similarly, most of the papers presented in Anthropology seminars relate to ethnographic accounts of health behaviour practices and functioning of local health practitioners. There is description, no analysis in terms of theory or policy planning. Even the textual great health traditions of India and China, namely Ayurved and Chinese Medicine have been discussed under ethno-medicine in 'Medical Anthropology' by Foster and Anderson. Actually, I discussed this matter with George Foster who accepted the argument, that textual medicine could not be termed as Ethno-medicine.

Instead of discussing the practices and knowledge of shamans and herbalists under ethno-medicine, it would be more appropriate to discuss under the conceptual framework of Little tradition and Great tradition enunciated by Robert Redfield. The interaction between Little and Great tradition in India is obvious since the classical texts are generalizations of the folk practices, as are evident in home remedies and kitchen medicine. Similarly, the concept of anatomy and physiology in Indian and other traditional systems of medicine discuss metabolism and immunity. The concept of *Shukra* and Ojas are the guiding principles about masculinity in patriarchal mind which hindered vasectomy programme in India culminating in Indira Gandhi loosing political power.

Medical anthropology is applied anthropology about health aspect of culture. It is now common knowledge that applied anthropology was rated low in anthropology. George Foster accepted that his teachers, Herskovits, Kroebar and Lowie had successfully inoculated him against the germ of applied work, since it did not contribute to anthropological theory. Foster countered this argument by the fact that much of culture change theory came from materials collected through applied anthropology. On the other hand, medical professionals made critical comments about the post-mortem evaluation of their programmes by anthropologists, instead of participating in implementing them. We are aware that after the Third World countries became Independent and aspired for welfare and development of the people, the expectations of leaders from intellectuals and academicians to contribute to the development process were high. In India, after the community development programme was embarked in 1952, which included the installation of institutional primary health care in rural areas, several anthropologists from Western countries came as consultants to design extension strategies in community development. Anthropologists and later, professional social workers, were called upon to educate the illiterate people to adopt agricultural and health technologies for their development. The conceptual variation between the acceptance of agricultural technology with visible results in few months as against the perceived or propagated results of modern science in medicine has not been understood even now. It takes time for the people to experience the effects of immunization or therapy in controlling epidemics and mortality which is different from the visible results of agricultural or engineering technology. For this reason, people prefer to follow time tested traditional therapies or practices, particularly in areas of maternal and child health. People have confidence that in the least, there would be no adverse effects. There are too frequent changing messages about the causation of cancer, or about transmission process of leprosy, therapeutic or disease causing factors in food and so on. It was argued that magic was being marketed in the name of science in such products as tooth paste or detergents. What AYUSH would advocate to consume is being marketed as herbal cosmetics to be applied to the body to improve skin complexion. The promotion of behavioural change communication (BCC) is considered as a magic pill to solve health and disease problems. Paradoxically, the over use of agricultural technology is probably creating an issue of farmer's suicides and the degradation of soil health. The technology of sonography has accentuated female foeticide.

We are aware that curative medical technologies from all systems of medicine have been accepted by the people, but not those in the preventive and promotive aspects which contradict the basic cultural norms and values. Female foeticide and low age at marriage of girls do not show any appreciable change for the better. Vasectomy continues to be unacceptable. Condom is not used in marriage as safe sex tool to prevent HIV. Condom is not used widely between a female sex worker and her frequent client, with whom an emotional relationship has developed. Cross-cousin marriage could be a preferred type in South, while it is branded as incest in the Hindi belt. Anthropologists understand the rationale of these behaviour patterns. We explain seemingly contradictory behaviour with the use of concepts of hard and soft core of culture backed by needs doctrine of Malinowski's functionalist theory. However, Health Education programmes having gone through the terminological change to Information, Education, Communication (IEC) seem to be asserting on Behavioural Change Communication (BCC) to which anthropologists are supposed to contribute. The whole paradigm of health care programme is to get the people to accept what is offered to them by medical model, to solve people's problems created by powerful bacteriological agents in the epidemiological triangle with the use of chemotherapy and vaccines. They want anthropologists to help them in social marketing of IEC and BCC among the lay people to accept and convince them as to how 'slight behavioural change of compliance' will solve the problems created by bacilli and viruses. People are blamed for drug resistance in TB or Leprosy for not adhering to regular treatment without looking at other contributory gaps about supply of drugs or confidence building, counselling or failure to communicate total information about the disease to the people.

The paradigms of health programme are medicalised, in many cases governed by distribution of medical products coming from the pharmaceutical industry. These programmes, therefore, do not address to people's concerns. For example, leprosy afflicted are concerned about social exclusion as a result of deformity, mutilation and ulcer. The control or eradication programme is concerned about identifying the bacillus and killing it. Since deformity is caused by nerve damage, anthropological perspective of priority medical research should be in the area of nerve damage in preference to drug research. HIV/AIDS conveys that HIV and AIDS are synonyms which they are not. Any counselling to HIV+ve person that AIDS could be postponed by pursuing healthy life style does not make any impact on the mind, since HIV/AIDS are presented as one single term separated by a slash.

The argument is that, medical anthropology should address the issues of policy planning significance, using anthropological theory and research tools. The strength of anthropological research lies in qualitative methods which answers the question 'why' to enable the quantitative numbers to communicate the process. (Mutatkar: "Medical Anthropology: Past, Present and Future" in *Explorations in Indian Medical Anthropology*, ed. Bhat, Joshi, Vijayendra: Vol. 1: 2013: 49-51).

III

Health is usually understood as absence of disease. In that sense, health is discussed as a therapeutic medical concept giving prominence to disease control programmes. Since disease control programme has a global perspective and linkage with the pharmaceutical industry and medical profession, it gets precedence over health prevention and promotion activities. India shares the global concerns of chronic, stigmatizing diseases such as Leprosy, HIV and AIDS and TB. The national health concerns relate to child and women's health. In India, we have inherited plural systems of medicine such as Allopathy, Ayurved, Unani etc. Besides, we have special issues about tribal health. Health and disease are also considered moral issues. A healthy person, and an elderly person who gets quick natural death are considered to be morally superior to those who suffer from chronic ailments and have to pray for death as release from suffering, if they remain bed ridden for a long time. A disease is, therefore, considered deviance from morality. Chronic diseases like leprosy, HIV and AIDS and TB are stigmatizing and get associated with the idea of sin, either in this birth or past birth.

Health matters have been considered as biomedical phenomena. However, people have varying beliefs and practices about personal body image, nutrition, causation of diseases, environment including plant and animal life, and fire and water. There are varying practices having a bearing on health which relate to dietary patterns, personal hygiene, mating patterns, child birth and child rearing, age and sex groupings, social regulations of interpersonal and group contacts, family relationships and occupation structures. These cultural beliefs and practices and many others make health a social-cultural phenomena.

All societies provide for sick roles since they cannot afford to lose the productive and role playing manpower through premature deaths or by falling victims to various diseases. Societies would obviously be more concerned with chronic, communicable diseases, but the efforts to control these could be constrained by the lack of evidence based traditional knowledge and experience about curability of such diseases in a society. People have experienced treatability of several communicable diseases by the use of allopathy, although the chronic ailments continue to be difficult to cure in a short time.

Health is an aspect of culture like economic, political, social and religious aspects of life. Culture being an integrated whole, all aspects are interrelated. In any traditional society, the integration is close knit, the static or equilibrium spirit overriding the dynamic nature of culture. Health aspects could be classified into softer or visible aspects such as treatment regimen of any sort, which provides relief from illness. Ideas about prevention and promotion of health and causation of illness are part of hard core of culture, which would fall in the area of belief. Cause-effect relationship about health and illness, therefore, fall in the areas of belief system. The plural treatment therapies, which may be herbal or of synthetic drugs in modern medicine, are guided by results. Magico-religious procedures are also followed in health, more so in tribal society, but not totally absent in the developed societies. There is no vacuum of knowledge or practices in matters of health and medicine in any society. People have their own perceptions of cause-effect relationship about disease and treatment, which may appear rational or non-rational. There are professionals in tribal society, generally referred to as Bhagats, Vaidu, Baiga or Gunia who have good knowledge of herbal medicine, besides some of them practicing magico-religious procedures. Tribal people have faith in these healers since they are a part of the kinship community and are always accessible.

Human communities are interested in health and disease cure of its members. In the animal world, sick are left to use environmental resources for recovery or die. Amongst human beings, members of the group attempt to restore sick person to health, to enable him to perform normal social role obligations. It is believed that in case of leprosy in the past, where recovery was considered impossible, the deformed sick were left to fend for themselves until leprosy colonies provided shelter to them. Community was to be protected from communicability of leprosy by sacrificing a leprosy afflicted family member by physical isolation and social exclusion. There was a separate church for leprosy afflicted in Munich (Munchen). Deformed leprosy beggars continue to be abhorred, although many amongst them are burnt up cases.

Medical systems have developed as a vast complex of knowledge, beliefs, techniques, roles, norms, values, ideologies, attitudes, customs, rituals and symbols; in short, a totality of health knowledge, beliefs, skills and practices of the members of every group. Briefly, a medical system embraces all of the health promoting beliefs and actions and scientific knowledge and skills of the members of the group that subscribe to the system. Every society has its own concepts of health, disease causation and health care. Usually, health is understood by lay people as a totality, perceived by appetite for food, body metabolism, good sleep, and body-mind vitality to perform social roles.

There can be conceptual difference between disease, a pathological concept and illness, a cultural concept. Usually, a person with disease is treated to cure his illness. In health sector it is necessary to use the services of herbalist medicine man and *Dai* for providing the services to the people. Their knowledge and skills could be updated for better results.

These observations have evolved from the ethnographic knowledge of tribal culture from fieldwork experience in anthropology. Ethnography in classical anthropology refers to the description of culture traits, patterns and complexes. In the era of planned, directed change, it is necessary to have the understanding of the interaction of macro-level policies and programmes with micro-level logistics rooted in the culture of the people. This is what Jawaharlal Nehru meant when he said that the change should be according to the genius of the people. It is, therefore, necessary to redefine the anthropological understanding of holism. Holistic approach can no more be limited only to the holistic and integrated understanding of the culture of an ethnic group. It should refer to the understanding of macro-micro and etic-emic dynamic interaction which could help to bring about sustainable cultural and social change.

Conceptually health care by the people at home, health care services provided by traditional local healers and private sector, and health care delivery by the government provide variety of paradigms. Gradually with the growth of medical education, private clinics by the doctors, but more so, private practice by experienced compounders, pharmacists, MPWs and RMPs became a common site in village India. The growth of AYUSH medical colleges did not necessarily increase the professional manpower pursuing AYUSH health care delivery, since both in public sector and private sector, AYUSH medical graduates mainly practice allopathy. However, all these developments led to a parallel National AYUSH Policy and establishment of AYUSH Department under Ministry of Health and Family Welfare. For the first time in India, AYUSH Ministry has recently been formed with independent authority. Hopefully, a single National Health Policy will emerge to project the vision of integration of plural medical systems which should benefit the common man.

IV

As there are plural culture systems, there are plural health and medical systems. In India, the health culture systems are Ayurveda, Yoga, Naturopathy, Unani and Siddha to which Homoeopathy and Tibetan medicine have been added with an acronym, AYUSH. Due to British rule and the development of modern science, allopathy or modern medicine or Western medicine has become the dominant medical system in health care of the people. More particularly the communicable disease control programmes are designed as per allopathy.

In spite of the resolutions to propagate Indian systems of Medicine in pre-independence days, probably due to influence of two national leaders, who were reputed physicians, Dr. Jivraj Mehta from Bombay (now Mumbai) and Dr. B.C. Roy from Bengal, allopathy got the position as Mainstream system of medicine after Independence. National Rural Health Mission (NRHM) has tried to co-locate all systems of medicine with little success. India may be the only country in the world with two official National Health Policies.

Why are we promoting AYUSH? We promote AYUSH because lay people, particularly in the villages are already following the principles and practices of AYUSH. They are using food as medicine, kitchen condiments as medicinal decoctions, plants and herbs, which are mentioned in AYUSH classics as of medicinal value. There are local indigenous herbalist professionals who treat people. They also supply herbal material to AYUSH professionals, and pharmaceutical industry. What people follow in their homes are the little or local traditions and what is given in the classic texts are the great traditions of the same health care phenomena. Only that lay people do not use the terminology of great tradition. They do not recite *samhita*.

In the people's sector in Indian homes, more particularly in rural homes, home based herbal remedies are being practiced as the first line of defence for common ailments. Kitchen condiments or flower-leaf offerings to deities at home are all of medicinal value known to elders in the family. Even the lady doctors from all systems of medicine follow traditional health practices when they become mothers themselves. People are aware about the health and medicinal value of different food products and their mixtures in diet. Nutritious food is offered to deities on ritual and ceremonial occasions, as per people's perception about nutritious diet which need to be offered to the ancestors and family deities. With increased demand for vegetables during ritual period for ancestor worship, the prices of vegetables sore high without the demand going down.

V

Development of the concept of welfare state has led the state to assume the responsibility of health of the people. Concepts of health, disease and treatment based on modern biology and modern medicine have created structures and organizations for healthcare delivery, as we witness them today across the world. Traditional medicine has been reduced to the label of alternative medicine, in developed world.

Community development programme in 1952 which was a major exercise in planned nation building in rural India had health as one of the prime components. Primary Health Centres were established as part of community development programme.

Anthropologists were called upon to educate illiterate communities to change their behaviour and attitudes, in order to accept modern methods of agriculture, health care and disease cure systems. Plethora of KAP studies indicated the research role of Anthropologists in documenting the baseline information and subsequent change. "India's Changing Villages" by Professor of Anthropology, S.C. Dube was one of the first books on community development. Anthropologists like Oscar Levis, David Mendelbaum, George Foster and Morris Oplar came as consultants in this process. The basic paradigm was that people needed to change their behaviour and comply with modern science and technology for their own development and for nation building. Traditional medicine was ridiculed as quackery and the concepts of hot and cold, and light and heavy were made a laughing stock, by those who could visibly show increased agricultural production with the use of modern agricultural technology of seeds, fertilizers, pesticides and irrigation. They could not and do not understand the varying paradigms of soft and hard aspects of culture.

The Western World is now shifting towards alternative medicine, as a consequence of side effects of scientifically produced drugs, and medical system monitored by insurance companies. People are tired of unnecessary and expensive use of diagnostic tools and techniques, in the absence of clinical acumen on the part of the physician. We are aware that after Independence, modern medicine has become the national health care system in India. Officially plural systems of medicine exist in India by way of medical colleges, research institutes, pharmaceutical industries, and Government departments in all systems. The Central Council of Indian Medicine, Indian Council of Medical Research, Medical Council of India and the like are expected to oversee medical education and research. However, the budgetary provisions and the infrastructure of public health care delivery system clearly indicates bias in favour of modern medicine. Indian Systems of Medicine (AYUSH) do not figure in Primary Health Centres, and if so, without the adequate supply of AYUSH drugs. AYUSH Health Centres function only as OPDs, having no public health functions. Allopathy and AYUSH run as parallel rails, never to meet. NRHM had an objective to bring them together through co-location, not yet with visible success.

VI

The Task Force on Mainstreaming of AYUSH systems in the Eleventh Plan has identified certain disease conditions for which there is overwhelming evidence of better cure in Ayurved, Unani, Homoeopathy, Yoga etc. which could be made available to patients as complementary or alternate therapy. Since majority of the health problems are at the primary level, there is need to increase the outreach of health care delivery at the village level. It will help if an AYUSH doctor is posted to look after a cluster of three sub-centres. There is a valid case for AYUSH module to be included in the MBBS course-curriculum. The central focus has to be on mainstreaming of AYUSH under NRHM, as recommended by the Task Force.

The Steering Committee on AYUSH for the Eleventh Five Year Plan had appointed a Working Group on AYUSH in Public Health under the leadership of a medical anthropologist, the author of this book. The group's observations as under and subsequent recommendations from the social science perspectives deserve consideration.

"AYUSH is the health aspect of Indian Culture and Society, historically evolved and used by the people without external support, with the use of local health professionals, traditions and indigenous knowledge and wisdom. AYUSH is expressed as Great Tradition in ancient books like Charak and Sushrut which evolved by conceptualizing the folk and little traditions of the common people based on empirical experience. The sustainability of AYUSH can be increased by promoting the interaction of Great and Little Tradition and through reinterpretations to suit the needs of modern times and by upscaling with the use of modern science and technology. Uniform standardized research methodology of AYUSH, not necessarily based on modern medicine, need to be evolved and systematic documentation need to be promoted. There is no conceptual conflict between the local health traditions practised by people and folk practitioners, and those practised by formally educated AYUSH practitioners."

"Plural systems of medicine have historically evolved in India. AYUSH systems are rated low and marginalized like the Scheduled Castes and Tribes (SC & ST). Without implementing the principle of Equity, historically marginalized AYUSH could not be empowered for integration. The advances in modern sciences such as physics, chemistry, botany and molecular biology etc. present modern medicine with more visible effects. There is no reason why these sciences and resultant technology cannot be used by AYUSH. State of the Art diagnostic tools and tools for measurement of health and disease according to modern science need to be available to AYUSH."

"Ideally, integration should be manifested in the integrated National Health Policy and the integrated NRHM document without special treatment or mention of AYUSH as one single point. Distinct National Policy and programmes of AYUSH, creation of a separate department of ISMH in 1995 and the vast infrastructure of AYUSH is an acknowledgement of the empirical realities created for the use of AYUSH for health care of the people, in the public sector, the position which AYUSH should have enjoyed as the mainstream health aspect of Indian culture."

"However, mere deployment of AYUSH personnel and medicines in the existing (Public Health) PHC and referral system, based on modern medicine geared to Western knowledge about health and disease management, and the markets flooded by modern pharmaceuticals, would not lead to functional integration. These systems are headed by modern health professionals at all levels who are ignorant about AYUSH and brand it as inferior or quackery or placebo" (December 2006).

The Steering Committee on AYUSH for the Twelfth Five Year Plan has made some recommendations which have direct link with the studies reported in this book. Research on folk healing practices as local health traditions or little traditions need to be undertaken. On lines of Ayurved Gram concept in Chhattisgarh, AYUSH gram in the public sector has been recommended which could link the AYUSH health centres with Panchayati Raj Institutions (PRI), Community Based Organizations (CBO) and Self-Help Groups (SHG).

Ethnographic studies have been conducted in Himachal Pradesh, Madhya Pradesh, Chhattisgarh and Maharashtra by collecting primary data from the villages as per protocol of study. The study of Rajasthan by SEDEM and other eighteen States by NHSRC have been cited. The studies conducted in twenty three States in India document the grassroots realities about health care by people, health care services, health care delivery and about the concerns of the people, paramedics and professionals.

VII

The National Policy on Indian Systems of Medicine and Homoeopathy (ISM&H), 2002 envisaged integration of AYUSH Systems into public health system and National Health Programmes, ensuring optimal use of the infrastructure of hospitals, dispensaries and physicians. Integration of AYUSH systems at all levels can strengthen the public health care systems and will create interest and faith in ISM&H and will facilitate people's access to natural, safe, friendly and time tested remedies. To make integration possible and to make it responsive to people's needs, restructure of the health care mechanism of AYUSH and public health system will be required.

The National Rural Health Mission (2005–2012) has been started to provide effective health care to rural population throughout the country to improve public health indicators and infrastructure. Reduction of neonatal, infant and maternal mortality, universal access to public health services, integrated comprehensive primary health care and prevention and control of communicable and non-communicable diseases are some of the main goals of the mission. It has key components like village health plans prepared by local village health and sanitation committees and panchayats and strengthening of rural hospitals for effective curative and referral care as per Indian Public Health Standards. It seeks to revitalize local health traditions and mainstream AYUSH into public health system. It also aims to regulate private sector including the informal rural practitioners to ensure availability of quality services to people at reasonable cost and promote Public-Private partnership for achieving public health goals. It seeks to improve access of rural people, especially poor women and children to equitable, affordable, accountable and effective primary health care. The Mission plans to undertake architectural correction of the health system to effectively handle increased allocations under the National Common Minimum Programme and promote policies that strengthen public health management and service delivery in the country.

Mainstreaming of AYUSH is one of the strategies under National Rural Health Mission the objective of which is to provide accessible, affordable and accountable quality health services to the poorest household in the remotest rural regions. It is known that AYUSH systems of medicines are well accepted by the community especially in rural and tribal areas. AYUSH medicines are comparatively safe, economical, easily available and can be prepared with locally available resources. Through the main-streaming of AYUSH component, the Mission seeks to revitalize local health traditions.

Mainstreaming of AYUSH is to be achieved under NRHM by mainstreaming AYUSH infrastructure, including manpower and drugs to strengthen the public health system at all levels through co-location of AYUSH doctors and facilities in PHCs, CHCs and District hospitals. Utilisation of services of AYUSH doctors after training and orientation towards providing advocacy, counselling and dissemination up to village level and promotion of AYUSH medicines at grassroots level in different national health programmes is envisaged. Important interventions aim at inclusion of AYUSH medications in the village level kit of ASHA, inclusion of AYUSH formulations in the supply of generic drugs provided at SC, PHC, CHC levels, appointing AYUSH MOs at single doctor PHCs and providing place for AYUSH practitioner and pharmacist at CHCs as per IPHS model. Total functional integration between AYUSH dispensaries and hospitals and general health care facilities under allopathic system is envisaged so as to make available the entire spectrum of AYUSH and Allopathy systems of health care to the public so that people can exercise their choices for treatment. This will help to lower maternal mortality, infant mortality and total fertility rates.

VIII

In this book, an attempt has been made to present the documentation of culture friendly and people centric AYUSH medical system as it is functioning in 23 States in India. Human development refers to the capacity of the people to make choices to improve their quality of life. Let the plural systems of medicine available in India be made accessible and affordable to people to enable them to make considered and selective choices for different sorts of health care needs as single therapies or plural therapies for the preventive, promotive and curative requirements.

3

STUDY DESIGN

Emic and Etic Approaches

Genesis and Road Map

As a follow-up action of Task Force Report of the Department of AYUSH for the Eleventh Five Year Plan, AYUSH Steering Committee of Planning Commission nominated a Working Group on AYUSH in Public Health, under the Chairmanship of Prof. R.K. Mutatkar. In consequence, one of the recommendations to appoint Commissioner for AYUSH equivalent to the status of Secretary was accepted in some States in India. The recommendation was made on the lines of ICDS model to be funded wholly by the Central Government.

At a meeting with Shri Shiv Basant, Joint Secretary, Department of AYUSH, Government of India, on 31st January, 2007, the Joint Secretary proposed a rapid study about the Mainstreaming of AYUSH in Health Care. This was followed up by about two hour discussion meeting with the Secretary Mrs. Aneeta Das and Joint Secretary Shri Shiv Basant at Delhi on 8 June, 2007 about the proposed study to be undertaken in the States of Himachal Pradesh, Madhya Pradesh, Chhattisgarh and Maharashtra in the context of NRHM, to be completed in about 6 months' time. The presentation of the draft project proposal was made at the Department of AYUSH, New Delhi on 2nd August, 2007, at a meeting chaired by the Secretary AYUSH, and attended by Joint Secretary, Advisers, Deputy Advisers, Assistant Advisors and Directors of the AYUSH Systems of Medicine. Dr. R.S. Arole, Padma Bhushan was also present who agreed to the suggestion of the Secretary, to be the Co-Investigator of the Study Project. The Secretary while summing up the discussion, made a specific suggestion—"The study should aim at making an exact assessment of what AYUSH is doing in health care delivery and what should be done for promoting the use of AYUSH systems by the masses."

Foundation for Revitalization of Local Health Traditions (FRLHT), Bangalore, convened a Workshop on AYUSH in Public Health at Bangalore on 8-9 February, 2008, whereby the format for formal grant application was handed over to Prof. R.K. Mutatkar by the Under Secretary Shri S.D. Sharma, who was representing the AYUSH Department. Formal sanction letter and the demand draft for the grant was received soon after in February 2008. A request was made to the Joint Secretary AYUSH to send letters to the respective State Governments about the Project which were personally collected by the Principal Investigator and dispatched towards the end of June 2008. In the meantime, a similar study was sanctioned to Society for Economic Development and Environmental Management (SEDEM), New Delhi, for study in Rajasthan, under the guidance of Shri Arun Shrivastava. There was also a discussion for similar studies to be undertaken in other States by National Health Systems Resource Centre (NHSRC), New Delhi, under the guidance of Dr. Ritu Priya, Professor at the Centre of Social Medicine and Community Health at Jawaharlal Nehru University (JNU) on deputation to NHSRC. Both the organizations were advised to follow MAAS research protocol by the Joint Secretary Shri Shiv Basant. The Department of AYUSH formally requested MAAS to function as national level coordinator for such studies on AYUSH in Public Health. However, it was decided to accept this responsibility after the MAAS Project of four States was completed, since the already approved budget for MAAS study had no budget line for discharging this responsibility. MAAS participated in the meetings in August 2008 to formalize the tools of research to be followed in all these studies. MAAS was also initially involved at the orientation workshop of the team of NHSRC study.

Himachal Pradesh Government represented by Dr. Rakesh Pandit, O.S.D. at the Directorate of Ayurved, was the first to respond to coordinate the project in his State. Dr. R.S. Arole and Prof. R.K. Mutatkar visited Shimla on 13-14 October, 2008 and met the Secretary of Health and other officials. They also made a brief field visit at Chiyog to see the AYUSH dispensary and meet the doctor and the Gram Panchayat members. This was followed up by Prof. R.K. Mutatkar visiting Dr. G.S. Badesha, Director of Ayurved, Chhattisgarh and Shri Mukesh Varshney, IAS, Commissioner of AYUSH, Madhya Pradesh Government at Bhopal. During this process, the field sites were selected in consultation with the respective Directorates of AYUSH and district level officials. Similarly, a team of four Research Assistants in each State was also selected as per recommendations of the Directors. Each State was headed by an Honourary Coordinator to supervise the work. Dr. Hemraj Sharma, an AYUSH Specialist in Ksharsutra Chikitsa was deputed by the State Government to help us in Himachal Pradesh. In Madhya Pradesh, Prof. A.N. Sharma, Head of the Department of Anthropology, Dr. H.S. Gour University, Sagar, and Prof. Mitashree Mitra, Head of the Department of Anthropology, Pandit Ravishankar Shukla University, Raipur, Chhattisgarh, volunteered to coordinate the project in the respective states. In Maharashtra, Prof. R.K. Mutatkar assisted by Dr. Shailesh Dalvi and Dr. Kalpana Mutatkar monitored the project which was mainly focused in the tribal areas.

After preliminary field work in all the States, the feed-back and study instruments finalization workshop was held at Pune during 27-31 January, 2009. The workshop was attended by all the State Coordinators and fourteen Research Assistants whereby orientation on Research Methodology was given to all the participants. All field sites were visited by Prof. R.K. Mutatkar and Dr. Robin Tribhuvan from Pune to monitor the data collection process. Draft State reports were presented at the State meetings at the Directorates and Secretariate (as detailed in Chapter 7). Presentation of the final draft report was made at AYUSH office, New Delhi on 3rd August, 2009 at a meeting chaired by the Secretary, Smt. S. Jalja and attended by the Joint Secretary, Directors and the Advisers, Deputy and Assistant Advisers of AYUSH systems in the Department of AYUSH. The Secretary in her concluding remarks offered Centre of Excellence: AYUSH in Public Health to MAAS. The meeting was attended by all State Coordinators of the Project, Dr. R.S. Arole and Shri Darshan Shankar, Director, FRLHT, Bangalore, and Adviser to the Planning Commission.

Research Methodology

Anthropological perspective of the study:

The study was planned according to anthropological perspective. Anthropology being the science of holistic study of man and his works, respects all cultures and all plural systems of health and medicine as they satisfy the basic needs of respective societies. It is the science of Medical Anthropology which studies health and plural medical systems, as all are functional for respective communities.

Originally, the study was to be aimed at assessment of mainstreaming of AYUSH systems under NRHM. It was, however, decided to sponsor the study by the Department of AYUSH and not under NRHM flagship.

To address the objectives as outlined by the Secretary, AYUSH, it was decided to follow the Emic approach for research. Emic refers to the insider's view of behaviour and practices. The classical anthropological model of ethnography of a single culture is designed by using the methods of participant observation and informal interviews. For focused ethnography such as about health care perspectives of the people, interview or observation guides are made to help as check list. Home remedies followed by the people in their homes as cultural traditions are best documented by emic approaches. Etic approaches refer to interpretation of behaviour and practices by an investigator by using more structured tools of data collection such as interview schedules and questionnaires. When people refer to the services rendered by health care providers in an institutional set up, such as at the Sub-centre, Anganwadi, Ayurvedic Health Centre or at the Primary Health Centre, etic approach is more suitable for data collection. The data tools followed by NHSRC and SEDEM in their field investigations are prominently belonging to the etic approaches, while those followed by MAAS in four States conform more to the emic approach. It is thus the combination of emic and etic, primary and secondary data, quantitative and qualitative data, that has helped to provide the ground reality of AYUSH utilization in 23 States in India.

NHSRC had initially planned to cover all States. However, Department of AYUSH had just then commissioned the Maharashtra Association of Anthropological Sciences (MAAS), Pune, to undertake a similar study of AYUSH services in four States, Maharashtra, Madhya Pradesh, Chhattisgarh, Himachal Pradesh, and the Society of Economic Development and

Environmental Management (SEDEM), Delhi, for a study in Rajasthan. In the discussion with the Joint Secretary Department of AYUSH, it was decided to coordinate the studies so as not to duplicate efforts and still provide an all-India picture. Tools were developed jointly by the NHSRC and SEDEM teams with constant communication by email of drafts of the various schedules at each stage to MAAS (NHSRC 2010: 13).

NHSRC and SEDEM objectives of the study were to focus more on mainstreaming of AYUSH under NRHM.

NHSRC study was aimed at providing an overview of the status of initiatives at mainstreaming AYUSH and revitalization of LHT' under NRHM as well as of the other services of the AYUSH systems in the public sector across all States. Some general issues for health services development and for strengthening of AYUSH services in particular were expected to emerge from this investigation, with special significance for implementation of the NRHM strategy. While the public services were the main focus, a few private facilities were also to be included to reflect their situation and utilization pattern.

In each state, one district was selected for the study. The district with the best services in the state, other than the district in which the state capital is situated, was selected. The 'best' was identified based on the number and level of existing facilities, as well as in consultation with the State department for its rough evaluation of their quality of functioning.

Within the district, 2 blocks were selected, one a well developed block and the other a backward block. All stand-alone AYUSH facilities in the block and one CHC, 2PHCs with co-location and 4 SCs were studied per block. Community perceptions were sought from the SC villages and through exit interviews at the selected facilities.

For exit interviews, 8-10 patients were to be included per institution, identified serially as they came out after consultation etc., was completed. If the institution had less than 5 patients/day, all were interviewed.

Any major private or NGO facility reported in the area was also included. At least 2 such facilities were to be studied per district. Any folk healer who had good popularity, as reported by the institutional providers or by the households, was also to be interviewed.

For the household interviews, 10 households were selected in each SC village. Identifying the major social groups (by caste, tribe and religion) and clusters in the village, an appropriate number of households in each was selected. For instance, if 5 clusters were identified, 2 households could be selected per cluster by a process of random selection (NHSRC 2010: 7-9).

The SEDEM study of Rajasthan about 'Assessment of AYUSH after Mainstreaming' comprised survey-sampling of AYUSH doctors, allopathic doctors, and out-patients. Gram Panchayat Pradhans were interviewed to elicit their views on healthcare problems and AYUSH. The study team also visited manufacturing facilities, herbal farms, and research centre to understand the constraints in production of quality medicines and formulations, supply of raw materials, and problems in conducting clinical trials.

The second part of the SEDEM study was part of national studies with NHSRC and the Maharashtra Association of Anthropological Sciences (MAAS, Pune, headed by Prof. R.K. Mutatkar). This part comprised of small sample but with in-depth investigations into integration problems under NRHM, documentation of patterns of uses of home remedies, local health tradition and patterns of use of allopathic facilities. The study team also interviewed ASHA and Gram Panchayat Pradhans (SEDEM 2010: Foreword).

The SEDEM research team adopted systems approach. The study covered medical facilities, elicited views of AYUSH and Allopathic doctors on a variety of issues including integration, village level issues in implementing NRHM, trends in the use of home remedies, and local health traditions. The study team also covered manufacturing facilities, herbal farms and research centre.

The data collection included sampling of AYUSH doctors (181), Allopathic doctors (105), exit poll of users (1111), and G.P. Pradhans (84). Data was collected on structured interview schedules from AYUSH and allopathic heads, gram panchayats, users of integrated facilities (patients) in accordance with an agreed data collection instruments developed jointly with NHSRC and The Maharashtra Association of Anthropological Sciences (MAAS) (SEDEM 2010: i).

Field Objectives of MAAS Studies

1. To understand the ground realities about preventive, promotive and curative health care from AYUSH or plural

systems of medicine in public, private, voluntary and indigenous sectors at institutional, professional, paraprofessional, community and household levels.

2. To assess the role of paramedics and traditional healers in the use of AYUSH in curative, preventive, and promotive health care.
3. To assess the training and IEC material needs for mainstreaming of AYUSH.
4. To assess the significance of plural therapy and cross-referrals between Allopathy and AYUSH streams.

Geographical Area and Population Selection

- Four States, namely Himachal Pradesh, Chhattisgarh, Madhya Pradesh and Maharashtra were selected for the study as per discussion with the Secretary and Joint Secretary. The response of the State Governments to the Government of India letter was very positive about the studies in their States. They expressed satisfaction that they would get the ground realities from the field in their respective States.
- Study area and population within the States was selected in consultation with the respective State Governments. State Government had to select one district in each State, 2 blocks in a selected district, 2 PHCs in each selected block, 2 sub-centres under each selected PHC and 2 villages under each sub-centre.

Table 3.1: State-wise selected areas: Four States

Sl. No.	*Unit*	*Himachal Pradesh*	*Chhattisgarh*	*Madhya Pradesh*	*Maharashtra*	
1.	District	Hamirpur	Bilaspur	Sagar	Pune Rural	Tribal 7 Dist.
2.	Blocks	2	2	2	2	9
3.	CHC/PHC	4	5	5	4	14
4.	AHC	3	3	2	2	—
5.	Homeopathy/Unani	1	—	2	—	—
6.	Sub-centres	4	8	8	—	19
7.	Villages	8	16	16	—	63

- The area coverage in Maharashtra was partly from rural and partly from tribal areas, from 9 blocks of 7 districts, where an intervention project on malnutrition, 'Adivasi Utthan Karyakram' (AUK) (Comprehensive and Sustainable Human Development of the Tribal People of Maharashtra) was being implemented by MAAS, funded by the state government.

- The organization of AYUSH health care delivery system from state to village level was studied in the four States along with the infrastructure available to deliver the health services. AYUSH health institutions were visited, meetings were organized and discussions held with health functionaries at various levels.
- Primary and secondary data was collected at the State level and from the field visits in the districts under study.
- Stake holders meetings were held in each of the four States at district and State levels. The meeting in Himachal Pradesh was most successful where health functionaries of various categories from public and people's sector discussed the issue of mainstreaming of AYUSH in public health care delivery system and recommended the interventions required, at organization and infrastructure levels to bridge the existing gaps.

Manpower Coverage for Data Collection

Responses from all sectors of population and health functionaries from the informal, indigenous, professional and paraprofessional sectors were studied. The study covered following sectors:

1. **People's sector** covered men and women from households, Baiga/Vaidu/herbalists, *Dai*/TBA, Village PRI representative, pregnant women and mahila mandals (women groups).
2. **Government sector**: Personal interviews/meetings with AYUSH health personnel and officers at state, district and block levels including health secretary and health minister as in Himachal Pradesh. Medical Officers (MBBS and BAMS), Paramedical personnel, namely ANM, MPW, ASHA/Mitanin, Pharmacist, Midwife, Anganwadi workers were interviewed.
3. **Private sector**: Pharmacist from pharmacy shops and private practitioners interviewed.

Table 3.2: Details of Geographical area coverage (As recommended by the respective State Government):

Sl. No. State	*District*	*Block*	*PHC*	*Sub centre*	*Village*
1. Chhattisgarh	Bilaspur	1. Pendra	1. Kotami	1. Kotami SC	1. Kotmikala 2. Dumdum
				2. Devaikhurd SC	3. Devarikhurd 4. Devarikala
			2. Navagaon	3. Navagaon	5. Jhaba 6. Bai Umrao
				4. Amadand	7. Sonbachharva 8. Jatadevari
		2. Marvahi	3. Dhobahar	5. Nimdha	9. Nimdha 10. Kasinwa
				6. Dhanpur	11. Dhanpur 12. Larkeni
			4. Sivani	7. Sivani	13. Badraudi 14. Devgavan
				8. Pandri	15. Dharhar 16. Ainthi
2. Madhya Pradesh	Sagar	1. Kesali	1. Sahajpur	1. Amoda	1. Bedar 2. Amoda
				2. Muhali	3. Muhali, 4. Saraivan
			2. Tada	3. Kevalarikala	5. Kevalarikala 6. Narayanpur
				4. Tada	7. Umariya, 8. Khaerikala

Sl. No. State	District	Block	PHC	Sub centre	Village
		2. Sagar	3. Dhana	5. Dhana	9. Samaramgad 10. Bandana
				6. Hilgan	11. Hilgan 12. Sallaiya
			4. Karbana	7. Karbana	13. Karbana 14. Muzgava
				8. Bamoharidodar	15. Bamoharidodar 16. Dugasara
3. Himachal Pradesh	Hamirpur	1. Bijhad	1. Saloni	1. Harsaur	1. Harsaur 2. Bhalat
				2. Jaulidevi	3. Batarli, 4. Baditar
		2. Nadoun	2. Barsar	3. Nara	5. Nara 6. Budain
				4. Gahali	7. Gahali 8. Nagareda
4. Maharashtra	Thane	Jawahar Mokhada	14 in 9 blocks	19 in 9 blocks	68 villages in 9 blocks out of 250 villages under AUK
	Raigarh	Karjat			
	Nandurbar	DhadgaonAkkalkuwa			
	Amravati	Dharni			
	Yavatmal	Zarijamni			
	Gadchiroli	Etapalli			
	Ahmadnagar	Rajur			

Table 3.3: Manpower coverage under the three sectors for primary data

Sl. No.	Sector	Individuals and Groups	States				
			Himachal Pradesh	Madhya Pradesh	Chhattis-garh	Maharashtra	
						Rural	Tribal
1.	Peoples' Sector	Households	214	165	180	32	499
		Mahila Mandal	4	—	—		
		Pregnant Women	23	—	—		
		Baiga/Vaidu/Herbalist	3	10	36	5	43
		Dai/TBA	9	24	31	4	39
		Village Head (PRI)	3	1	2	2	—
2.	Government Sector						
	(A) Doctors	(I) PHC Doctors (MBBS)	4	4	4	2	4
		(ii) Ayurvedic Doctors	9	2	4	3	13
	(B) Para-Professionals	(I) ANM	13	8	7	6	22
		(ii) MPW	—	—	2	—	—
		(iii) ASHA/Mitanin	N.A.	10	92	4	49
		(iv) Pharmacist	2	—	—	—	—
		(v) Mid-wife	1	—	1	—	—
		(vi) AWW	16	25	35	6	63
3.	Private Sector	(I) Doctor	1	2	14	3	4
		(ii) Chemist	3	6	2	—	—

* The data collected with the quantitative and qualitative research tools and techniques has been presented in the book in narrative, tabular form, also as Annexures.

The Selection and Training of Study Team

The study teams were selected to study the ground realities about AYUSH in four States. The study teams consisted of Research co-ordinators from Pune, State coordinators and research assistants from the States of Himachal Pradesh, Chhattisgarh and Madhya Pradesh.

One State supervisor was identified in each State who was to monitor the study. In Madhya Pradesh and Chhattisgarh the Heads of Anthropology Departments of Universities were identified. In Himachal Pradesh a senior AYUSH Medical Officer was assigned by the State AYUSH department to help the study team.

The supervisors (co-ordinators):

1. Prof. A.N. Sharma, Prof. and Head, Department of Anthropology, Dr. Harisingh Gour University, Sagar, Madhya Pradesh.

2. Prof. Mitashree Mitra, Prof. and Head, Department of Anthropology, Pandit Ravishankar Shukla University, Raipur, Chhattisgarh.
3. Dr. Hemraj Sharma, Senior Medical Officer, Department of AYUSH, Himachal Pradesh.
4. Dr. Shailesh Dalvi, Pune, Maharashtra, Dr. Kalpana Mutatkar assisted Prof. R.K. Mutatkar, in Supervision of the project.

As per the recommendations of respective State coordinators, four research assistants (two male and two female) were selected in each of the three States of Madhya Pradesh, Himachal Pradesh, and Chhattisgarh, and one in Maharashtra. In Madhya Pradesh and Chhattisgarh the research assistants were post-graduates in Anthropology. In Himachal Pradesh, the field investigators were graduates from local communities. In Maharashtra, part of the data collection was undertaken by the project assistants of a tribal project (AUK).

In January 2009 all research assistants from three States with their respective State coordinators received orientation training at Pune, for three days, for understanding the study objectives as per terms of reference. The research tools to be used for data collection, the process documentation for the expected outcomes were standardized. Before coming to Pune, the research assistants had lived in the villages selected for study in their respective States to explore ethno-medical beliefs, practices, maternal and child health related practices, local health traditions, health seeking behaviour, and the nature and role of traditional medical practitioners. The teams presented their preliminary field experiences and findings at Pune. This pre-training exposure to the study area was very useful for study as it helped the researchers to understand the project objectives and the methods of data collection in a better way to achieve the expected outcomes. In anthropological field training, it is advisable to jump in the field without too much literature survey so as not to get biases which could limit or mould field investigation to what has been given by other authors. The general knowledge of the area and the people, gained in preliminary field visit helps to compose the research tools in a more meaningful way for focused ethnography.

Eleven interview guides-*cum*-semi-structured schedules prepared for data collection were finalized during the training with inputs from the four State coordinators in view of variations of language and practices in the four States. Research assistants' initial exploratory fieldwork proved useful in planning the details of study design. The tools were prepared in Hindi and Marathi. The project proposal, terms of reference, the components of NRHM mission document were also translated in Hindi.

Research Tools and Methods of Data Collection

During the period of three months the research team gathered primary as well as secondary data. The secondary data was mostly quantitative and was gathered from various reports from State and District level AYUSH offices, while primary data was mostly qualitative and was documented by research team during field visits with the help of following tools:

1. **Interview guides:** Eleven Interview guides-*cum*-schedules were prepared for interviewing health functionaries from the three sectors, i.e. people's sector, government sector and private sector. These interview guides were used for interviewing ASHA/Mitanin, *Dai*/TBA, Baiga/Vaidu, Anganwadi worker, ANM, Medical officer PHC/AYUSH Health Centres, Pharmacists, Chemist shop, and private practitioners. Household survey and village profile formats, and formats for getting information about infrastructure of health institutions namely PHC, Subcentre, and AYUSH health centres were used.
2. **Case studies:** Important and striking features of a particular study were documented in details in the form of case studies, e.g. of *Dais*, Baiga, CHC and PHC etc.
3. **Observations:** While collecting information using interview guides certain observations about health institutions were documented to support the qualitative data. Since the research assistants stayed in the villages with the families, real life participatory and non-participatory observations were recorded.
4. **Daily Diary:** Following the classical anthropological field method, daily diary (log) was maintained about movements, meeting and discussions held with people.

5. **Focus Group Discussions:** Informal interviews with peoples' groups such as pregnant and lactating women, mahila mandals, paramedical workers, women from households to discuss a specific common subject helped to get deeper insight and information about the ground realities of common practices.
6. **Body mapping as participatory technique:** was used while interviewing *Dais* and to know about their understanding of fetal formation and growth.
7. **Social mapping:** technique was used in a group of key informants to draw a village map giving details about the boundaries, roads, important landmarks, facilities including health care in the village as perceived by them.
8. **Consultative meetings at district headquarters:** were arranged for getting feedback from AYUSH administrators and doctors at district and state level. Various issues related to mainstreaming of AYUSH were discussed. The information regarding existing deficiencies in infrastructure, staff positions, drug supply, the strengths of AYUSH, people's demands of health care, the issue of co-location etc. were documented along with their recommendations.

Presentations of draft State reports were made at the Directorate and Secretariate levels. In Himachal Pradesh, presentation was made to the Hon. Minister of Health and Ayurved at Shimla with participation by Secretary Health, and Director AYUSH. Final presentation of draft report was made at the Department of AYUSH, Government of India, New Delhi to the Secretary, Joint Secretary, Directors, Advisers of all AYUSH systems on 3 August, 2009.

Limitations of MAAS Study in Four States

While the strength of the study lies in the total co-operation of the respective State governments at all levels in the collection of data, and total dedication of the young field teams, uniformity of data is lacking in the States. Despite Himachal Pradesh team not formally trained in anthropology, supervised by a senior AYUSH clinician, the ethnography of verbatim reporting of community responses as written in their diary note books has been excellent. Madhya Pradesh and Chhattisgarh field teams were composed of fresh postgraduates in Anthropology, who stayed in the villages for considerable period. In Madhya Pradesh, structured questionnaires were used with statistical analysis of data to supplement the qualitative data. Chhattisgarh team has given more qualitative data focusing on Mitanin (ASHA) and Baiga (Herbalist). In Maharashtra, there are no exclusive Ayurvedic Health Centres in comparison to the other three States. Since a tribal project was being simultaneously implemented, there have been more details about tribal herbalists and *dais* (TBA).

Due to administrative delay of effective communication about the project from the Department of AYUSH, Government of India to respective State governments, there was pressure to meet the deadline of completion of the project.

With anthropological, ethnographic bias in the MAAS project, the gains about data from the community overtook the studies about NRHM objective of mainstreaming of AYUSH. Keeping in view the readership, the theoretical perspective of relationship of health and culture particularly in the traditional communities has been repeatedly emphasized. The co-location was discussed but was not visible in operation in the four States at the PHC level except in Maharashtra which was not designed as per NRHM requirements. Co-location was still at the planning and coordination level in the respective health departments. There appeared to be reluctance at the level of allopathic institutions to accommodate AYUSH facilities in their buildings or premises.

However, despite the logistic variations between the studies conducted by MAAS, SEDEM and NHSRC the data brings out the totality of AYUSH systems as they function as health care system and as practised as cultural tradition by the communities.

4

PEOPLE SECTOR
Health Care

Introduction

Indian systems of medicine, namely Ayurved, Unani, Siddha, and Yoga and Naturopathy are being used by people across India since ages. Homoeopathy is being used across India in homes on a wide scale. People have been taking treatment from Vaidyas and Hakims who were practicing Ayurveda and Unani systems with medicines prepared from medicinal plants, herbs, spices and condiments used in cooking and some animal products. Minor ailments were taken care of by frequently used home remedies which got popular as Grandmaa's medicine. The knowledge of these remedies got passed on through generations and even now the people have faith in these remedies as they are affordable being cheaper, accessible being available at home and without side effects, being of herbal origin and not chemical synthetic compounds produced by modern pharmaceutical companies. The home remedy practices referred as little traditions of community were later on compiled by masters like Charak, the great Ayurved physician and became the basis of Ayurved system and text. Similar processes have been in vogue in Unani, Siddha and other Asian systems of medicine.

Allopathy or so called modern medicine is of Western origin and had its entry in India during colonial rule initially for health care of British Army focusing on malaria. It gained upper hand in formal health care system after Independence while the Indian systems got sidelined. The National Health Policy was formulated in 1983, revised in 2002 without giving due consideration and place to Indian traditional systems in health care delivery. Allopathy prospered in formal health care set up at Government level. Having realized the inadequacy to reach the entire population, a separate administrative structure, Department of Indian Systems of Medicine and Homoeopathy was established in 1995 and a separate National ISM&H policy was also designed in 2002. The Department was renamed as Department of AYUSH in 2003. This Department as a part of Government of India's Ministry of Health and Family Welfare, has brought under one umbrella all non-allopathic systems including local folk practices or ethno-medicine, formally called as local health traditions. Recently in November 2014, a Minister with independent authority has been appointed for AYUSH, providing strength to the Department.

In spite of the development of huge network of Allopathy and AYUSH systems with the related infrastructure and manpower, it is observed that these systems need to work complementing each other as no single system is found to be capable and perfect enough to manage the health issues and disease burden of varying nature. The great contribution of modern medicine is in the decline of communicable diseases and related mortality and morbidity due to vaccines and therapy. However, with economic development and related prosperity there is the emergence of non-communicable diseases which are lifestyle disorders. To manage and treat these disorders the Indian systems of medicine have strengths which need to be used in national health care system. NRHM has one of the components for mainstreaming AYUSH in its Mission document. However, mainstreaming of AYUSH should effectively mean incorporating AYUSH under each component of the Mission.

The study of People's Sector has explored the community level ground realities about people's practices in regard to curative, promotive and preventive health care at house hold level as home remedies. The different types of ailments treated by family members with the help of commonly available herbs and kitchen spices as medicines is documented under the title of home remedies. The part of plants used as medicine, form in which it is administered and the process of preparation is also documented. Information about people's perceptions and knowledge about AYUSH and Allopathy health care systems, their problems and needs about access to health care, and their health seeking behaviour is documented.

The views and recommendations of community, local health providers, e.g. Baiga/Vaidu/herbalist and *Dai*/traditional birth attendant for promoting AYUSH in mainstream health care highlight the need for increasing community awareness about strengths of AYUSH, training of health workers in AYUSH and need for integrated health care by giving equal weightage to plural systems, encouraging cross referrals and positive attitude towards AYUSH from allopathy health care providers in order to improve the existing health care facilities at community level.

People's Preferences: AYUSH *versus* Modern Medical Care and Self-Referral Practices

Through the household visits and community based FGDs with men and women, people's understanding and perceptions about different systems of health care, their knowledge, experiences, choices and preferences for a particular system as regards ailments could be understood. In Himachal Pradesh people seemed to have clear understanding about limitations of Allopathy system usually referred to as modern medicine and the risks of modern drugs by way of side effects. Ayurved was referred as 'our own system'. On the basis of their knowledge gained through observations and practices of elders in their families, people were practicing home based care as first line of treatment for common ailments.

Allopathy based health care was approached if home based care failed to give relief or in situations of emergency or for surgical interventions. Access to public sector health centres such as sub-centre, primary health centre, rural hospital or ayurved health centre depended on the distance and severity of illness. If accessible by time and transport, ayurved health care at AHC was preferred first.

In Madhya Pradesh after the first line of health care with home remedies, the next choice of referral was for the local herbalists. ANM at sub-centre and Ayurved dispensary of the government were preferred as the third choice depending on the nature of ailment and accessibility. The local health functionaries like ASHA, Anganwadi worker also seemed to follow the same route of referral services for themselves and their families. ANM and AWW many a times bypassed local herbalist, unless he was a specialist for some specific ailment like piles or paralysis. ASHA in her own case, however, consults herbalists like other village women. Mitanin (ASHA) in Chhattisgarh has close links with herbalists, locally called as Baiga.

Household Level Health Care: Practice of Home Remedies

The people's sector was covered to understand the home based and community based local health care practices as home remedies for treatment of common ailments by utilizing kitchen condiments or common local herbs found in the backyard, in village surroundings or nearby forest. A retired ANM in Himachal Pradesh had remarked that *"Her kitchen was her home dispensary"*.

Through household visits in the study area the home remedies which were commonly used as a first line of treatment for symptomatic relief of common ailments like cold and cough, constipation, fever, vomiting, diarrhoea, piles, toothache, headache, body ache, joint pains, skin diseases, injuries, weakness, piles were documented. Treatment known to people for problems like jaundice, paralysis, gynaecological problems, diabetes, urinary stones, snake bites etc. was also noted. The remedies included kitchen condiments, common herbs and specific locally available medicinal plants. The names of the herbs and medicinal plants used by people were documented in their local language and later scrutinized by Ayurved doctor for equivalent botanical names (Details in Annexure).

Majority of the people got information about home remedies from the elderly in the family (54%). 55 per cent reported that they could identify medicinal herbs. About 15 per cent persons reported availability of medicinal herbs in the compound of the house, about 20 per cent reported from the village and about 18 per cent reported availability in the forest, in the neighbourhood. 80 per cent reported the kitchen condiments such as turmeric, asafetida, fenugreek, garlic, onion, jaggery, mustard seeds, cumin seeds, coriander seeds, cinnamon having medicinal properties.

About the method of using the herbs, 83 per cent reported that they mixed the herbs in tea, milk or took with water. Among the multiple answers, 35 per cent prepared decoction (*kadha*), 24 per cent used for massage mixed with oil and 17 per cent roasted and 27 per cent grounded the herbs for consumption. Household processing of medicinal herbs is common. Thus methods of administration of home remedies varied from simple powders, paste, decoctions, local applications, fomentation, inhalation etc.

The names of the herbs used for common ailments in four States are given as Annexure.

Table 4.1: Home-Remedies: Home made preparations, single or mixed herbs

Sl. No.	Common Ailments	States						
		Chhattisgarh		Himachal Pradesh		Madhya Pradesh		Maharashtra
		Herbs	Product	Herbs	Product	Herbs	Product	Herbs
1.	Cough	23	30	19	17	17	13	21
2.	Cold	23	30	20	07	14	11	10
3.	Fever	13	09	11	06	07	04	10
4.	Constipation	19	13	13	14	13	09	—
5.	Vomiting	04	02	08	05	11	11	13
6.	Diarrhoea	20	16	12	07	17	11	13
7.	Headache	15	12	11	06	12	12	7
8.	Jaundice	13	07	02	01	11	07	—
9.	Body Pain	09	06	15	09	12	07	14
10.	Joint Pain	09	06	06	03	07	09	14
11.	Weakness	14	07	04	02	18	12	6
12.	Injury	14	12	04	03	07	09	8
13.	Gynaec problem	06	05	01	01	14	10	04
14.	Bone setting	06	04	05	02	07	01	03
15.	Skin Disease	11	08	03	02	13	13	05
16.	Toothache	05	03	—	—	07	04	—
17.	Renal Calculi	01	01	01	01	—	—	01
18.	Paralysis	02	02	—	—	—	—	—
19.	Diabetes	01	01	02	02	—	—	—

Source: Research Team's field investigation.

Views of Villagers

The local villagers said that though there are a number of government health schemes going on in the villages, they have not been implemented properly and the villagers are not benefiting from it. According to them the reason behind this is the lack of quality and number of the local staff and the lack of proper facilities. They said that the health workers do not visit the villages regularly and when they do visit they do not have adequate or proper medicines with them. They also complained about the lack of transport facilities in case of emergencies and deliveries.

The villagers informed that they used home remedies for common ailments and were satisfied by the results. They said that in present times it is difficult to find the herbs and plants easily due to the effects of deforestation. It takes time to search for the ingredients and prepare the formulations and hence gradually people are using them less and less, as the allopathic medicines are easily available and are faster acting in comparison to the Ayuvedic medicines. They said that they used Ayurvedic medicines for chronic illnesses and when the allopathic medicines did not provide a cure.

Many of the villagers have maintained herbal gardens and kitchen gardens for preparing Ayurvedic medicines and homemade formulations. The villagers still follow traditional health practices and demanded the easy availability of good quality Ayurvedic medicines.

NHSRC Studies about People Sector

NHSRC report on 'Status and Role of AYUSH and Local Health Traditions' under NRHM is very useful and strong in terms of the validation of community knowledge about home remedies in regard to some disease conditions, mother and child care, medicinal plants and food items as medicine. Major findings on these subjects have been reported as under:

(A) Home Remedies

In 11 of the 18 States, 80 per cent or more households reported use of home remedies. In 5 States 40-80 per cent use was reported, and in 2 States below 20 per cent use was reported. Generally, across the States the responses for diseases like cough and cold, diarrhoea, anaemia, constipation and joint and back pain were high. Six States show above 80 per cent households giving a positive response for usage of home remedies for one or more of the specified conditions, 4 above 60 per cent, 6 almost 50 per cent, and only one State had responses in the range of less than 40 per cent The conditions where no home remedies are commonly used, were similar across the States such as emergency conditions, accidents, heart diseases and surgical conditions, to name a few.

Validation of the Home Remedies

We had asked specifically for home remedies for a list of 20 conditions. We are presenting the analysis of only 3 disease conditions here as illustrative of the general patterns; the diseases being among the commonest conditions covering the communicable, non-communicable and nutritional categories, have been included—diarrhoea, anaemia and diabetes. Three conditions denoting promotive and preventive action have also been included; MCH, malnutrition and convalescence. As a general finding, 70-95 per cent of the reported home remedies in use under the above mentioned categories were validated in all States by the AYUSH references.

Validation of Home Remedies for Specific Conditions

- *Diarrhoea*: For diarrhoea, the validation across States was quite high in the range of 83-100 per cent. Some of the common remedies mentioned across the States were lemon juice with sugar and salt, buttermilk, *Ajwain, Pudina,* black salt, coconut water and raw banana, to name a few.
- *Diabetes*: For diabetes, the home remedies mentioned by the households were found valid in the range of 72-100 per cent across States. *Karela* (bitter gourd), *Jamun, Methi* and *Neem* were most commonly mentioned across the States.
- *Anaemia*: For anaemia, the remedies mentioned were valid in the range of 71-98 per cent across the States. Some of the common examples found valid as per Ayurved and Siddha across the States were beetroot, dates, *Munakka,* banana, *Curry Patta, Anar* (Pomegranate), *Masur dal,* milk and papaya. Duck soup, fish and chicken soup, were amongst the common remedies mentioned in Nagaland.

Other than the above, most of the preparations mentioned as home remedies like castor oil in constipation, *Neem* in skin diseases, and pepper with honey and *Tulsi* for cough and cold, are age-old known remedies fully validated by Ayurveda. The laxative action of castor oil, immunity enhancing effects of *Tulsi,* and anti-infective properties of *Neem,* are now accepted with modern scientific evidence also.

In Odisha, for 20 types of health problems 84 types of home remedies were used. Validation of all these show that 80 types (95.2%) were as per Ayurveda's principles and references in classical texts.

(B) Use of Home Remedies for Mother and Child Care

Specific questions about use of LHT for mother and child care in different stages elicited responses showing a high usage for RCH issues specifically under the headings of home remedies for healthy pregnancy, safe delivery, healthy lactation and health of the baby.

Home remedies were used for healthy pregnancy by 80-98 per cent of the households in the High Focus States, except Odisha (58%) and Karnataka (5%). In the Non-High focus States, it ranged from 0-80 per cent; West Bengal, Kerala, Delhi and Haryana in the range of 50 per cent and above; Tamil Nadu almost 20 per cent; and Andhra Pradesh not reporting its use. The proportion of users went up further for safe delivery and lactation.

Even for safe delivery, home remedies were reported to be extremely well used by the households, e.g. as many as 11 States reported more than 60 per cent use and the rest in between 10-50 per cent. Generally, all the High Focus States (districts) reported high use with an exception of Odisha at 50 per cent, and Jammu & Kashmir at 10 per cent. The better-off States like Kerala, Punjab and Tamil Nadu also reported high use.

As many as 10 States reported 80-95 per cent households using home remedies for healthy lactation; 4 States reported 40-70 per cent use, and the rest 4 States reported less than 40 per cent with Jammu & Kashmir as less as 22 per cent.

Kerala did show over 90 per cent use for baby's health. In all the MCH users, Kerala was a high user state among the Non-High Focus States (38-90%), with Andhra Pradesh a high user for all, other than the safe delivery. Odisha comes out as an intermediate user reporting State (50-90%), with Jammu & Kashmir being consistently among the lowest users (5-45%).

Validation of Home Remedies for MCH

Under this category, home remedies were asked for four specific conditions; healthy pregnancy, safe delivery, healthy lactation and baby's health. The remedies were found valid in the range of 70-86 per cent across States.

Use of *Amla*, milk products, eggs, herbs, massage with *Til* oil, as well as Yoga (Uttarakhand) were mentioned in the States for ensuring safe delivery, massage and mother's milk for baby's health, and use of jaggery and ginger preparations pre and post-pregnancy are some of the examples quoted for mother and child health as home remedies, which find mention in the texts as well.

In all the age groups, food items right from cereals/pulses/ green vegetables to milk/dates/meat, all are considered important; jaggery, honey, dates, pulses and milk are also recommended items under AYUSH for daily nutrition. As many as 62 items were mentioned as home remedies as multiple responses by the respondents and all of them are valid as per Siddha principles.

(C) Validation of the Medicinal Plants

The medicinal plants mentioned by the households were verified by their botanical names validated by the contemporary compilations from classical texts. Almost all States found 100 per cent validation. Overall the community's awareness about medicinal plants was found validated in the range of 80-100 per cent with all the names mentioned by the households found in the classical references, e.g. *Tulsi* was validated for botanical name *Ocimum Sanctum*. Similarly, for plants like *Neem, Ashoka, Vasaka,* Aloe vera and *Giloy*, botanical names as well as classical validation was done. All States had *Tulsi* and *Neem* as commonly mentioned plants by the households.

(D) Awareness of Medicinal Uses of Food Items

Specific questions were asked about the medicinal uses of food items that they know about. Out of 18 States, 13 States gave 100 per cent responses on the awareness about food items with their perceived medicinal properties, namely Odisha, Jharkhand, Nagaland, Sikkim, Uttarakhand, Jammu & Kashmir, Delhi, Tripura, Punjab, Haryana, Tamil Nadu, Assam and Andhra Pradesh. All the households in these 13 States had long lists of usage of such food items. Two States out of the remaining 5 States, namely, Manipur and Bihar, gave over 90 per cent responses on the awareness of food items. West Bengal showed more than 80 per cent response; whereas Karnataka reported 50 per cent use; and Kerala a mere 10 per cent.

Apart from plant-based items, many food items with animal, mineral or sea origin were also part of the food items mentioned by the households. For example, use of chicken soup, dog meat, red meat and eggs for general weakness; use of raw rock salt, cooking in iron utensils for "increasing blood" (anaemia), and use of fish, cod liver oil and frogs (Nagaland), were found respectively across the States. Food items mentioned showed community specificity in terms of their geographical and cultural background.

Validation of Food Items as perceived by the households.

The validation of community knowledge about medicinal value of foods was largely verified by the texts, from 75-86 per cent items were validated across the States. Apart from plant-based items, many food items with animal, mineral or sea origin were also part of the food items mentioned by the households.

Among the food items mentioned, many items were for digestive disorders, for respiratory infections, or as nutritional supplements. Food items were mentioned for use in arthritis, diabetes, renal stone, asthma and worm infestation. It was interesting to see more than one medicinal property mentioned for a food item by the households, e.g. ginger for cough and cold as well as for digestion, which were all valid as per AYUSH principles.

(E) Community's Knowledge of Medicinal Plants and Medicinal Value of Foods

The knowledge was validated in all 18 States. More than 75 per cent of home remedies used for diarrhoeal disease, anaemia and diabetes, as well as in convalescence and maternal and child health (MCH) conditions, were validated across the States. This is generally indicative of the strength of people's knowledge and its links with the indigenous systems suggesting that it should be the base to build upon as a positive resource rather than being neglected or even denigrated, as often implied in the general Information, Education and Communication (IEC) messages and health providers' communications. This also implies that the people's knowledge can further be strengthened and updated as per AYUSH scientific episteme for larger prophylactic and therapeutic use. It can also contribute to the strengthening of content of the AYUSH systems.

Validation of Community Knowledge

Community knowledge was validated in Tamil Nadu using Siddha texts and principles since that was the most commonly used textual form of traditional medicine in the State. In West Bengal and Tripura, Homoeopathy was the most commonly available AYUSH system, but since we were validating knowledge of medicinal plants, medicinal value of foods and home remedies, we used Ayurved as reference, as we did for the remaining 15 States where Ayurved was predominantly in use.

It highlighted the fact that the local health traditions are ecosystem and community specific, yet they are closely allied to the codified systems of AYUSH, forming the folk roots of AYUSH. It also throws light on the relevance of community knowledge which is an accumulation of experiential knowledge coming from diverse sources and systems. It suggests that people's knowledge and practice can be the starting point for planning and strengthening health care and that the research in AYUSH should cater to validating and strengthening this knowledge in development of the system and taking it forward (NHSRC, 2010).

AYUSH Rajasthan Study by SEDEM

Of the 105 Allopathic doctors interviewed in Rajasthan from district hospitals, CHCs, and PHCs about 44 per cent reported use of home remedies for self and family. About 64 per cent would not prescribe home remedies to their patients and 36 per cent allopathic doctors would not prescribe AYUSH line of treatment to their patients.

Some of the common home remedies reported by doctors are based on holy basil, turmeric, ginger, black pepper, honey, hot milk, *ghee*, lemon, garlic, clove, clove oil, salt water, ginger tea and *neem* leaves in various forms (2010: 37).

This compares well with the lady doctors from all systems of medicine following traditional maternity practices based on Ayurved or Unani or Siddha when they become mothers themselves.

Mother and Childcare—Role of *Dai*/Traditional Birth Attendant (TBA)

Traditional maternity practices at household level for pregnancy care, for easy delivery and postnatal practices after delivery and during lactation and the role of *Dais*/TBAs as support system for health care of mothers and newborn across the four States were documented.

It was observed that traditional practices for Mother and Child Health had strong community base being rooted in societal culture. The home based practices about care of women during pregnancy, delivery and postnatal period and lactation had variations depending on the culture and local health traditions but were based on scientific Ayurveda principles. These practices prescribed by mothers and mothers-in-law or grandmothers are actually the Great Traditions enshrined in the classic texts of Ayurved, and other texts of Unani or Siddha.

In general, postnatal care for 40 days which includes rest, massage with medicated oil, diet and nutrition supplement are followed. Neonatal care from birth to 28 days included massage with medicated oil, cord care, keeping the baby warm of which 10 days are essentially massaged by *Dai* followed by family care. Infant-care like massage with oil, bathing, breast feeding is generally followed for one year. Special diet is provided for improving lactation up to 6 months.

Mother and Child Care Practices in Chhattisgarh, Madhya Pradesh, Himachal Pradesh and Maharashtra

The household practices in all the four States are largely common with slight variations in regard to care during pregnancy, birthing practices and rituals, gifts received by the *Dai* (TBA) and about weaning practices. The research team studied mother and child care practices in all the four States. The findings of the same are highlighted in the case studies given below:

- *Pregnant Women:* Pregnant women start seeking advice from a TBA from 1st month itself. They eat normal food during pregnancy, but after delivery take;
  - (i) *Toor dal* Soup
  - (ii) *Gud ladoos* (Dry fruits bound in Jaggery)

(iii) Cow milk/*ghee*

- *Birthing Practices and Rituals*
  - ➢ Majority, i.e. over 90 per cent of the deliveries are conducted at home by the TBAs.
  - ➢ Umbilical cord is cut by a blade.
  - ➢ *Brasica juncea* (Sarson) oil is used to massage the new mother and child.
  - ➢ *Chhathi* ritual is observed to name the new born.
  - ➢ The period of observing this ritual varies from one tribe/caste to another depending on the economic status. Among the Bhaina and Oraon tribes "*Chhathi*" is conducted between 15 days to 2 months. These poor tribes are unable to get money. Whereas among the Gonds the ritual is performed on the sixth day by majority of them.
- *Gifts received by the TBA:* The TBA receives Rs. 50 to 100, liquor, food, 10 kg rice, 3 types of pulses and wheat in some regions.
- *Actions taken during critical situations:*
  - ➢ TBAs refer difficult cases to PHCs or CHCs.
  - ➢ Call ANM or Doctor for help.
  - ➢ Blow air into the mouth of the new born.
  - ➢ Clean the baby with warm water.
  - ➢ Put oil on the fontal bone of the head.
  - ➢ Warm the baby with carom seeds (*ajwain*) put in a make-shift cloth-sack (*potli*).
  - ➢ Among the Gonds a new mother rests for 12 to 25 days, but among the Bhaina and Oraon (poor tribes) she resumes her household duties within 7 to 10 days time.
- *Weaning Foods:* Weaning foods are introduced from 5th or 6th month. Smashed rice, *dal* and glucose biscuits are given, to the child. In some areas the ritual of introducing weaning foods is known as '*dana phunkna*'. The paternal aunt, fathers' sister (*phupi*) of the new born chews raw rice grains and blows them on the mouth of the child to mark the beginning of introducing weaning foods. Prior to this ritual yet another important ritual, namely '*mundan*'—shaving of the first hair-takes place. The child is made to sit on the lap of the '*phupi*'. A towel is spread on the lap of the paternal aunt and a barber shaves the hair of the child.

The aunt then collects the hair and puts into a cloth. The parents of the child put the hair in a holy river. On this day the child, the barber, the TBA receives gifts in cash and kind from the paternal aunt, the parents, the grand-parents and relatives. Women who deliver in the hospital perform *'Chhathi'*, *'Mundan'*, and *'Dana Phunkna'* after coming back home.

Birthing Practices and Rituals in Himachal Pradesh

- In addition to common practices as followed in other States, there are minor regional variations.
- Contrary to rural areas of Chhattisgarh and Madhya Pradesh wherein 90 per cent of the deliveries are conducted at home; in rural Himachal Pradesh 60 per cent rural women prefer to go to CHCs and private maternity hospitals. In Himachal Pradesh people are better off economically as compared to rural inhabitants of Madhya Pradesh and Chhattisgarh. It was observed that among most families at least one person works on a salary basis in the Government set-up.
- 'Punjab' ritual is observed to name the new born on the 11th day.
- The period of observing this ritual varies from one community to another depending on the economic status.

The role of *Dai*/TBA as regards her duration of stay with mother, the nature of her skilled services to mother and newborn child especially during first week of postnatal period was explored. The special diets and nutrition supplements traditionally prescribed and used for promoting lactation and recovery after delivery and the practices for newborn and infant care were also documented as in Table 4.2. What has been presented in the table are only some examples.

It was observed that traditional practices about oil massage to mother and newborn with medicated oil, providing specially prepared highly nutritious food supplements to mothers for promoting lactation and health recovery for minimum one month after delivery and early initiation of breast feeding are widely

Table 4.2: Health Care practices about Mother and Child Health in 4 States as reported by families:

Sl. No.	*Delivery Practices and Care*	*States*			
		Chhattisgarh	*Himachal Pradesh*	*Madhya Pradesh*	*Maharashtra*
1.	*Dai's* help	10 days	12 days	6 days	5-15 days
2.	For easy delivery	Drinking Hot Black tea or liquid decoction, Warm milk, tea of Jaggery, Warm *khichadi*	Reduced Diet. Milk, Dates (*Chuare*)	Cow's Urine	Decoction of black pepper and cumin. Put root of Calotropis plant (*Rui*) on scalp
3.	After Delivery	Massage by Mustard oil	Massage by Ghee or Sesame oil	Massage by Medicated oil	Massage by coconut oil or *mahua* seed oil.
4.	For Lactation	Dry fruit + Jaggery *ladoo* Black Gram (*Udad Dal*), Raw Papaya, Milk, Bargad tree extract.	Pipli boiled with milk and Dry fruit—Jaggery *ladoo*—Clarified butter (*Ghee*), *Suji*, Almond (*Badam*), Cashew Nut (*Kaju*), Dates *Kishmish*, Jaggery, Coconut, Black Pepper boiled with milk and Dry fruit.	Asparagus (*Satavar*) with milk, Earth worm cooked in milk and Jaggery.	Asparagus (*Satavar*) roots, Chattany made up of Earthworm, Ginger, Garlic, Black Pepper Rice with Sesame chutney. Prawn curry fortified with earthworm extract. *Ladoo* made up of Common cress (*Ahaliv*)
5.	Breast Feeding	1-3 Hrs. after birth	2-3 Hrs. after birth	½ Hr. after birth	½ Hr. after birth
6.	Weaning Food	After 5-6 months Porridge	After 4-5 month	5-6 months	After six months
7.	Massage of baby	Medicated mustard oil– 1 yr.	Sesame/Mustard Oil 3 Yrs. Cow's Clarified Butter, *Zau* Varya, Nutmeg, Fennel Seeds, Dry Ginger, Saffron (*Kesar*)	Medicated mustard oil—1 yr. *Ubatan* of Turmeric	*Mahua* oil, *Til* oil, Coconut oil,
8.	Recovery after Delivery	Dry fruit, *Dry* ginger edible gum, jaggery *ladoo*	Dry fruits, Clarified Butter *Ladoo*, Milk, Green Gram Pulse (*Mung dal*), Coconut, Dry Ginger, Kamarkas, Black Cardamom, Fennel Seeds, Clarified Butter Milk *Gudkatira*	Jaggery *Ladoo*, *Harira*, *Daliya* and Green Gram Pulse (*Moong dal*), Milk	Fenugreek (*Methi*) *Ladoo*, Dry fruit *Ladoo* and *Ladoo* made up of Common Cress (*Ahaliv*)

followed. It is to be noted that *Dai* support was available in all the States during the crucial first week of neonatal period during which there are more risks to newborn babies and there is a need to have experienced person's help for neonatal care as well as for initiation of breast feeding and recovery of mothers from exhaustion of childbirth. This observation suggests strengthening and updating of *Dai's* skills.

In Himachal Pradesh 50 per cent of deliveries are home based. There are no maternity services offered at any level from AYUSH practitioners working in Ayurved Health Centres. A post of *Dai* as one of the staff members for each AHC is officially sanctioned by Department of AYUSH throughout the state for provision of midwifery services covering 1136 AHCs. However, there is a shortage of trained *dais* and large number of vacancies are to be filled. Due to shortage of other manpower in AHCs, the appointed *dais* sometimes have to work as attendants or pharmacists for dispensing drugs and helping medical officers to run the clinic.

Recently in the developed countries there is a growing demand for home based safe deliveries and minimum hospital stay. In U.K. the pregnancy, delivery and postnatal care including newborn care is entirely managed by midwives under the National Health Service with backup facilities of the specialists and the hospital care in cases of emergency.

In 9 blocks of Maharashtra under the tribal project, 383 *Dais* were trained in their respective areas with 3-4 rounds of training sessions. The training was imparted by experienced trained senior women health workers/*Dais* from Dr. Arole's CRHP, Jamkhed. Besides teaching them safe delivery practices, proper newborn care and use of herbal material for common problems was also taught to them. Special training was focused on identifying risk factors in order to refer difficult cases to a hospital. Training in birthing practices was also provided to women volunteers who were not *dais*. A *Bhil* tribal woman who conducted 25 safe deliveries after such training narrated her experiences to the Bhil Tribal Minister for Tribal Development in Maharashtra on a public platform.

To promote the concept of institutional delivery in the village community, *Dai* hut was constructed in villages where experienced trained *dais* were available for conducting delivery under sanitary conditions. For lactating women to improve lactation and weight of infants, food supplement–*Sattu* (Baked Wheat + baked Bengal Gram *dal*) fortified with Ayurvedic herbs *Shatavari, Ashwagandha, Pipali* and *Jeshtamadh* was given up to 6 months with very good results validated by increased weight of children.

Dais: Traditional Birth Attendant, Madhya Pradesh

From 16 villages of Sagar and Kesali block 24 *Dais* were interviewed. The *Dais* were mainly from lower caste. *Dais* are skilled to take care of minor problems and conduct deliveries safely. They got the training from their mothers-in-law. They can identify risk signals and timely refer the cases to hospital.

In the opinion of Kamalbai and Jirabai from Kharikala village of Kesali block, in hospitals women cannot receive care and food prescriptions and restrictions (*parhej*) which they provide, and so normal deliveries should be conducted at home, and only difficult cases or having serious problems should be referred to hospital. They use oil for lubrication of vagina to expedite delivery in cases of problem. Kamalabai knows neonatal care and importance of keeping baby warm, and early breast feeding within an hour of birth. She receives some cash money for her delivery work, or up to 5 kg of wheat.

Gendrabai from Narayanpur described traditional post-natal care of mother. The mother is given massage with groundnut oil medicated with garlic, *ajwain* and asafetida. Mother is given perineal fumigation with *ajwain* to prevent sepsis and early recovery of perineal region.

Discussions with *Dais* revealed that in their work, experience is important and based on the strengths of their experience, they work as *Dais* and manage situations which even doctors may not be able to handle. The experience comes from elderly women. *Dais* are from Dhanak community.

GROWTH OF FOETUS: A CASE STUDY-1

Gorabai Kallu Bansar: Madhya Pradesh

Gorabai: The T.B.A.

Gorabai Kallu Bansar, a traditional birth attendant, aged 65, illiterate, a member of Dhanak Caste, resident of Kevalari Village, of Kesali block in Sagar district—Madhya Pradesh, narrated her perception of the formation and development of foetus. Gorabai has an experience of 53 years of working as a T.B.A. and has conducted over 6000 deliveries, i.e. 113 per year in 4 villages of Kesali block.

Although Gorabai was trained at Sagar in 1999 and in Kesali CHC during 2002 for seven days, twice, she believes that her traditional methods of conducting delivery are best. Her knowledge of pre and post-natal care and birthing practices are amazing. Throughout her career as a T.B.A. not a single child died, while conducting delivery. She may have referred 100 difficult cases of delivery to CHC Kevalari and Sagar. She may have accompanied 80 cases to the hospital or CHC. A dedicated midwife says out of the 6,000 babies she delivered, she must have saved lives of 1000 children. She feels bad for two still born children, who she had to tactfully pull out to save the two mothers.

Formation of Foetus

On enquiring, how a foetus is formed, Gorabai said male inserts semen into the vagina of a woman, a bit of it enters into the uterus through a soft tube; the rest is wasted, as it comes out. This bit which enters into the uterus meets with bit of water released by the woman. This white fluid gets converted into warm red blood. This is live and moving blood, i.e. "*Jinda aur Phataknewala Khoon hota hai.*" This is how new life is created in the womb of a woman. On enquiring, how twins and triplets are formed. She laughed and said, "Some couples who have extra sexual power produce more and powerful semen and water than normal couples. When more semen enters into the womb there are chances of having twins or triplets." She added that she never conducted delivery of twins and triplets. The womb of woman which produces twins and triplets is very strong, said Gorabai.

Development of Foetus

Gorabai was given a paper to draw and show the stages of development of foetus. While drawing simple diagrams to demonstrate the growth of foetus, she furnished following informations from an emic perspective:

Preparation for Delivery

Gorabai stated that when a woman is in labour pain, she is made to lie down on a blanket or quilt. Hot water is kept in a container. Pieces of clean clothes to wipe the child are kept ready. A blade to cut the umbilical cord is kept. Groundnut oil is also needed for delivery. A pillow or a folded blanket is kept under the lower back of the woman just above the buttocks.

The Process of Delivery

The posture of a delivering woman is such that her head points towards east, while her parting legs are towards the west. Gorabai said that mother earth, the Goddess of fertility who is to the west on the opposite direction of the sun must see the child first.

The woman in labour is asked to relax. Gorabai then positions the foetus by holding the stomach of the woman with hands by gently pressing the sides. Gorabai applies ground nut oil on the opening of the vagina. "*Mitha tel mahila ke ander bharte hai, taki sharir ka muh chikana ho our bachchaa bahar aye.*" The oil accelerates the process of delivery.

As soon as the baby is out, it is cleaned with a cloth dipped in warm water. Gorabai also cuts the umbilical cord and ties a cloth on the naval of the baby. The baby is cleaned with hot water and warmed with *ajwain* (*Ajwan ki Sikai*) in a cloth bag (*potli*). The baby is then wrapped in a cloth and kept on the left side of the mother so as not to miss the heart beats and warmth of the mother.

Gorabai then cleans the new mother with wet cloth dipped in warm water. The next important task is to remove the "spoilt blood"—"*ganda khoon*" from her body through the vagina. Gorabai holds the stomach of the woman and removes the blood out by gentle massaging the stomach downwards. The "*Mahewari Khoon*", i.e. menstrual blood which is in the mother's body for nine months is removed, so, as to cleanse the woman. One should massage from the sides of the stomach or else the uterus is affected.

After an hour the new mother "*Chhivari*" is asked to feed the baby. Gorabai who has undergone training in Sagar and Kesali blocks says that the "colostrums milk"—"*Pahala Dudh*" is good for the new born baby. In case of cuts on the linings of the vagina, she applies *ghee* prepared from cow's milk mixed with turmeric. If stitching is required, an ANM or doctor is summoned.

Treatment of Umbilical Cord

The umbilical cord and placental waste "*Nal*" and "*Var*" is buried in the ground and on that fire is burnt, so, as to destroy it. Gorabai said, "if the umbilical cord gets into wrong hands, it can be used as a black magical means to hurt the new born and the mother."

When Does the New Mother Eat?

Gorabai's reply to this question was after five to six hours, she is given "*Gud ke ladoo*" also called "*Harira*" the ingredients of the *ladoos* are:

(i) Cashew nuts – (*Kaju*)
(ii) Dry grapes – (*Kismis*)
(iii) Almonds – (*Badam*)
(iv) Dry Ginger – (*Sunth*)
(v) Dry Coconut – (*Sukha Kopra*)
(vi) Dates – (*Chhuvare*)
(vii) Peanut crush – (*Mung phalli ka chooran*)
(viii) *Ghee* prepared from cow milk
(ix) Jaggery – (*gud*)
(x) *Makhana* – (Fruit of lotus flower)

The above ingredients are bound together with *ghee* so as to make round balls called "*gud ke ladoo*" or "*Harira*" The new mother is given one or two *ladoos* soaked in hot milk, twice a day. This diet, says Gorabai produces healthy breast milk.

Simultaneously, "*Khairi ka Pani*", i.e. hot decoction of *Khair* (*Acacia catechu*, fam. Minogeae) twigs are given to the woman so as to relieve her of pain and also cleanse her blood and digestive system. This hot water is given to her for 15 days after delivery thrice a day. In case, she wants to have warm water, tea or milk the new mother can have it.

The Ritual of *Pachhi/Saur Uthana*

Pachhi means five; *saur* means dirt/dirty or pollution and *uthana* means to pick up. On the fifth day the T.B.A. cleans/washes all the dirty clothes of the new born and the mother, massages and bathes both of them, she smears the house with cow dung so as to cleanse the house of the effect of the menstrual blood and its impurity.

Gorabai is not allowed to touch the child and the mother from the sixth day. Knowingly or unknowingly, if she touches either of them, they are bathed to purify themselves. From sixth day onwards, a *barber* wife looks after the baby.

The Ritual of *Chhathi*

Chhathi means sixth. On the sixth day the new mother is given regular food, i.e., *Dal*, Rice and vegetables. She, however, refrains from eating heavy, chilly hot and hard food, such as chilly chicken, meat, fish, dry fish etc.

(a) **Gifts received on the occasion of *Chhathi*:** Gorabai the T.B.A is given Rs. 100, 10 kg wheat, 2 kg pulses, a *sari* and food for five days for following services to the new mother and child.
   - Preparation for delivery.
   - Conducting delivery.
   - Cleaning the mother and baby.
   - Cutting and burning the umbilical cord.
   - Massaging, bathing and warming up the new born for five days.
   - Advice on diet and medication etc.

(b) **Naming ceremony:** A "Pandit" (religious priest) is called to name the baby. "The priest is usually a brahmin," said Gorabai. The baby has two names, first given by the *pandit* and the second one given by the paternal aunt (*Phupi*) of the new born. The name given by the *Pandit* is entered in school records.

***Mundan*:** Hair Shaving ritual.

Depending on the economic ability of the family "*Mundan*" first shaving is performed after a month, two months or even within a year's time "*Nayi*" (Barber) is summoned to shave the hair. He is given Rs. 30 to 100 for his services. The first shaved hair is put in a river or stream.

Weaning Food

A baby is given weaning food after 6 months. In fact since birth not much water is given to the baby, except in summer, when it is hot. The belief that prevails is water should be taken only after food; hence, the baby starts drinking water after the introduction of weaning foods. Foods like rice porridge, smashed rice and *dal*, biscuits etc. are given as weaning foods after six months.

Who takes over from T.B.A.?

A question was asked to Gorabai, as to "Who takes over baby care services from you after five days?" She replied, "*Khavasan*" (Barber's wife). A *Khavasan* massages and bathes the baby for a month or two. She receives Rs. 100 to 200, 3 kg wheat flour, *ladoos*, food and a *sari* for her services.

Difference between a Still Born and Living Child

According to Gorabai a living child in the womb, i.e. "*Jinda Bachcha*":

- Is warm ("*Garam hota hai*").
- Moves in the womb.
- One can feel his heart beats.
- He plays ("*Pet me khelta hai*").

Whereas a Still Born, i.e. "*Mara Hoova Bachcha*"

- Is cold ("*Thanda hota hai*").
- Does not move in the womb.
- One cannot feel his heart beats.
- He does not play ("*Pet me khelta nahi*").
- *How do you remove still born?*
- Gorabai puts her hand in the vagina to remove the dead foetus. She says after informing the family members about the still born, she removes the baby within 10 to 15 minutes

so as to save the new mother. Gorabai said she has removed only two still born children in her life time.

- **What methods are employed if a baby has breathing problems?**
  Sometimes immediately after the delivery a baby has breathing problems.
  During such times Gorabai uses following methods:
  - ➢ She quickly cleans the baby's face, mouth, eyes, ears and chest with a cloth wet in warm water.
  - ➢ She then blows air in the mouth of the new born (*hava phukte hain*).
  - ➢ Once the baby starts breathing, she taps the baby on his legs, once the baby starts crying, she knows he is out of danger.
  - ➢ Then, without wasting much time, she cleans other parts of the baby's body.
  - ➢ She then rubs the palms, legs and chest of the baby with "Camphor" Oil. She says, *"Bachcha Chikta hai" aur "Rota hai"*, i.e. he sneezes and cries. These are indicators of smooth and normal breathing. The baby is wrapped in a warm cloth and made to lie on the left side of the mother's chest. Gorabai says the baby feels safe, when he hears his mother's heart beats.
- **Is there special oil for massage?**
  Yes, replied Gorabai. I see to it that half a litre massage oil is ready before the baby is born. She said, "Half litre ground oil is heated. Then smashed garlic, carom seeds (*awjain* powder) and asafetida (*hing*) are put in it. Three ingredients are boiled in the oil and left to cool. The oil is then sieved in another container." Gorabai said, "Garlic, *ajwain* and *hing* have heat in them, which keeps the baby warm." The "*Khavasan*" (Barber's wife) also uses the same oil to massage the baby.
- **Belief about colostrum milk**
  Colostrum milk *"Pahela dudh, bache ke liye achchha hota hai"* is good for the baby, said Gorabai. I see to it that the new born is given this milk immediately. If for some reason the new mother does not get breast milk, cow's milk is given to the baby immediately.

- **Diet after delivery.** A new mother must eat "*Gud ke laddoo*" or "*Harira*" as they are nutritious and produces healthy breast milk. She can eat rice, *dal* and *roti*, but should avoid:
  - Chilly hot food.
  - Fish, dry fish, meat (heavy food).
  - Cold food, cold water etc.

    Consumption of such food leads to diarrhoea, digestive disorders, cold and cough among infants, said Gorabai.

    The infant, however, must feed on mother's milk for six months at least. Weaning foods can be introduced after six months.
- **Diet during pregnancy**

  There is no special diet given to a pregnant woman during pregnancy she eats normal food, works normally till the ninth month.
- **Rest after delivery**

  "In the rural areas a woman's role in the economic activities of the family is crucial", says Gorabai. She is like a "hearth" which needs to burn ("Work") constantly for the survival of the family. Hence, after 7 to 15 days a woman gets back to her normal working life.
- **Have you stopped using disposable delivery kit?**

  Yes, said Gorabai, I have never used it before. My mother-in-law who taught me the art of conducting delivery never used it. My daughter-in-law, who is also a T.B.A. in Narayanpur never used it. We believe our traditional practice is best. We did receive D.D.K. in 1999 from Sagar, but never used them.

How is the Knowledge of T.B.A.s Transmitted?

Gorabai said, "I learnt from my mother-in-law and so have I transmitted to my daughter-in-law. The knowledge must remain in the village, hence a daughter-in-law is chosen not daughter. Daughters get married and go to another village."

Himachal Pradesh

Seven *dais* were interviewed in depth in Hamirpur district in

Himachal Pradesh. They had received training at CHC Barsar. They received *dai* kit, but no orientation about herbs or Ayurvedic medicine. Pregnant women start reporting to the *dai* from third month of pregnancy. *Dai* refers critical cases to hospital.

Dai advises consumption of green leafy vegetables and fruits during pregnancy. For eleven days after delivery, *dai* stays in the house of the woman. During this time, she administers oil massage to the new born baby and her mother and washes their clothes.

A traditional *dai* Mahanti Devi, age 80 years, with 50 years of *dai* experience of 1500 labour cases has narrated her knowledge about foetal growth.

DEVELOPMENT OF FOETUS: A CASE STUDY-2

Mahantidevi, a traditional birth attendant, aged 80, illiterate, a member of Brahmin caste, resident of Harsaur village, in Bijahar block of Hamirpur district, in Himachal Pradesh, narrated her perception about the development of foetus. Mahantidevi has an experience of 40 years of midwifery practice. She has conducted over 800 deliveries. She did not undergo any training at the PHC or CHC.

- **Care of the new born**
  - TBAs take care of the new born minimum for 11 days. The baby is given massage, bath and medication by the TBA.
  - Colostrum milk is given to the new born after 12 or 24 hours.
  - Cow or buffalo milk is given if the baby cries.
  - The baby is made to sleep near the mother's left side, so, that he does not miss the mother's heart beats.
- **Care of the new mother**
  - A new mother is made to fast for 5 to 8 hours, for it is believed that her body should be cleansed internally.
  - In rural areas of Himachal Pradesh, a new mother is given only cow or buffaloe milk, wheat porridge (*daliya*), *Dal* soup and rice +green *moong dal* (*Khichdi*), for 10 days. However, on 11th day a ritual captioned "Punjab" is conducted to name the baby. From the 11th day onwards the new mother is given normal food.

Mahantidevi was given a paper to draw and show the stages of development of foetus. While drawing simple diagrams she demonstrated the growth of foetus. She furnished following information from an emic perspective.

Other Practices

Nutritious Ladoos: The new mothers are given *laddoos* called "Sund" after 11 days. The rural folk believe that the ingredients in the *laddoos* contribute to production of healthy breast milk. These ingredients are as follows:

1. *Mung dal*—lentil (pulse)
2. *Badam*—Almonds
3. *Kaju*—Cashew nuts
4. *Chhuvare*—Dates
5. *Ajwain*—Carom seeds
6. *Sonth*—Dry ginger
7. *Kamar*
8. *Kas*
9. *Magh*
10. *Pista*—Pistachio
11. *Desi ghee*—locally prepared *ghee*
12. *Haldi*—Turmeric powder

The local people believe that turmeric powder cures joint pain of the new mother and purifies blood. The ingredients in the *laddoos* are classified as hot food that gives strength to the lactating mother; relieves weakness, reduces pain and produces healthy breast milk.

- To purify the blood of the new mother, powdered dry ginger, smashed dates and jaggery is mixed with milk and taken.
- During the ninth month a pregnant woman takes warm milk daily in the evening with *ghee*. They believe this promotes the smooth delivery of the baby.
- A trained T.B.A. keeps following articles ready before the delivery.
  - Towel
  - Weighing Balance
  - Scissor
  - Hot water

- Soap
- Brush
- Sheet
- Blade
- Clean cloth
- *Sarson/Til* Oil
- *Dori* (Thread)

Mahantidevi believes that number eight is inauspicious and hence majority of children delivered during the eighth month die. On enquiring "what is the impact of iron tablets on the foetal growth?" Mahantidevi replied: "Most pregnant women take iron tablets".

According to another *dai,* Manshadevi, age 80 years, illiterate who conducts about 25 deliveries in a year for the last 40 years as social work, does not charge any fees. In case of risk of difficult labour, she refers the woman to a hospital at Galod or Hamirpur. According to her, many women go to hospitals these days and the incidence of caesarian operations is on the increase. Poor people who cannot afford hospital charges continue to invite her for labour. After delivery, the new mother is given wheat porridge with milk, and a mix of rice and green gram pulse (lentil) '*khichdi*'. Milk is given thrice a day. *Chapati, moong dal* without green skin and rice is also provided. This kind of easy to digest food is given for about 4-5 months. *Semolina porridge* fortified with dry fruits is given for gaining strength. Seasame oil or cow *ghee* whole body massage is given to the new mother. On the eleventh or thirteenth day, ritual for the baby is performed. Baby may be weighed in grain/food which is given to *dai.*

Dai/Traditional Birth Attendants (TBA): Chhattisgarh

Thirty one *Dais* were interviewed out of which 10 were trained and 21 untrained. 10 were tribal women and rest were non-tribal. Tribal women were from Gond, Bhayna, Oraon, and Dhulia tribes. Others were of Panika, Ghasiya, Yadav, Lohar and Chamar caste. *Dais* age group ranged from 45 to 80 and their experience ranged from 15 to 60 years. Most of them were illiterate. Only 7 were educated up to primary level.

87 per cent deliveries were home deliveries and 12.78 per cent were hospital deliveries. 44 per cent were conducted by *Dais*, 27 per cent by nurse, 20 per cent by relatives, 3 per cent by Chamarins and only 5 per cent by doctors. This statistics is important for policy

planning about training coverage required not only for known *Dais*, but also training women who are not labelled as *Dais* but are in need of training for safe delivery practices. 99 per cent reported the use of new blade to cut the umbilical cord. *Dai* conducts the deliveries but cord cutting and cleaning of room or clothes is done by lower caste women from Chamar or Ghasiya caste. *Dais* who were trained received delivery kit only once after the training. *Dais* could manage retention of placenta or save the baby in adverse situations.

After delivery women fast for a day. They are given medicines from Baiga herbalist to relieve pain followed by food. They have their own practices after delivery. 73 per cent reported initiation of breast feeding within 1 to 4 hours after birth. Prohibiting eating of sour things and green vegetables in diet after delivery was a food taboo practiced in all the households. 6 per cent informed starting of supplementary food to infants by 4 months of age but 100 per cent started that by 6 months. There was no difference in this practice for male and girl child. ANM demands Rs. 500 to 700 for delivery if called at home and also in PHCs. So many women prefer *Dai* and home delivery. *Dais* have been complaining that their traditional services of maternity and neonatal care are being passed on to inexperienced ASHA. For institutional delivery, even ASHA does not get any honorarium unless she maintains good relationship with ANM and AWW. Even if a *dai* takes a pregnant woman for institutional delivery, ASHA gets the honorarium which is denied to a *dai*.

DEVELOPMENT OF FOETUS: A CASE STUDY-3

Raniyabai Shriprasad Pirwar, a traditional birth attendant, aged 55, illiterate, a member of Gond tribe, resident of Devrikala village, in Pendra block of Bilaspur district, Chhattisgarh State, narrated her perception about the development of foetus. Raniyabai has an experience of 20 years of midwifery practice. She has conducted over 800 deliveries. She did not undergo any training at the PHC or CHC.

- **Care of the new born**
  - ➢ TBAs take care of the new born minimum for twelve days. The baby is given massage, bath and medication by the TBA.

- ➢ Colostrum milk is given to the new born after 12 or 24 hours.
- ➢ Honey, cow's milk or jaggery water is given if the baby cries.
- ➢ The baby is made to sleep near the mother's left side, so, that he does not miss the mother's heart beat.

- **Care of the new mother**
  - ➢ A new mother is made to fast for 24 to 48 hours, for it is believed that her body should be cleansed internally.
  - ➢ She is given bamboo shoot vegetables, with rice, *toor dal* soup, and dry fruit jaggery *ladoos* for production of healthy and quality breast milk.

Raniyabai was given a paper to draw and show the stages of development of foetus. While drawing simple diagrams she demonstrated the growth of foetus. She furnished following information from an emic perspective.

Raniyabai believes that number eight is inauspicious and hence majority of children delivered during the eighth month die. On enquiring "what is the impact of iron tablets on the fetal growth?" Raniyabai replied:

- A pregnant woman vomits.
- They don't feel like taking Fe tablets.
- They believe the heat in the tablets causes abortions.
- Foetus enlarges and delivery becomes difficult.

Dai/TBA Recommendations from Chhattisgarh

- They want to work in hospitals.
- Trained *dais* want refresher training.
- They want themselves to be attached officially with ANMs so that they can help in deliveries.
- Untrained *Dais* need to be trained by PHCS and AYUSH personnel.
- Delivery kit to be supplied regularly and monitored.
- Many *Dais* expressed their desire for incentives in cash or kind.
- *Dais* were interested in getting training from Government sector and suggested to include information about

Table 4.3: Growth of foetus: Summary of Three case studies

Sl. No.	*Month*	*Status of Foetal Development*		
		Madhya Pradesh Gorabai	*Himachal Pradesh Mahantidevi*	*Chhattisgarh Raniyabai*
1.	First	Living blood which is formed as a result of mixing of white male semen and female water. This blood moves. (*Khoon Phatakata hai*).	A bag of blood is formed.	The foetus is in the form of thick blood.
2.	Second	Starts becoming thick, but is red in colour	The blood starts becoming flesh.	The blood starts becoming flesh.
3.	Third	The red thick blood becomes flesh, weighing 200 gms. "*Dosau gram gath banata hai.*"	Flesh starts getting shape and form.	Real flesh is formed.
4.	Fourth	Flesh enlarges. "*Gath badti hai*".	Heart beats begins in the fourth month.	Head, hands, legs and eyes start forming.
5.	Fifth	Hands, legs and head is formed. It is soft though.	The baby starts playing, i.e. turning/ playing.	Heart beats start. ("*Dil put put karata hai*").
6.	Sixth	Baby starts moving and heart beat can be prominently heard. "*Bachcha hilne lagta hai or dil ki dhadkan sunai deti hai*".	Weight of the baby increases.	Hands and legs become separate.
7.	Seventh	The baby starts kicking and walking "*Lat marta or chalta hai*".	Dangerous for the baby, hence check-up is necessary.	Baby starts playing and turning. ("*Bachcha khelta hai aur ghoomata hai*").
8.	Eighth	Starts moving his hands and legs. "*Hat pair chalane lagta hai*".	Fully formed baby starts turning.	Skin colour becomes red.
9.	Ninth	Fully formed baby turns and rolls in the womb. "*Ghoomta-Phirta hai.*"	Baby is fully formed and is ready for delivery by the end of nine month.	Baby starts getting hair and is perfectly developed for delivery.

Source: Research Team's Field Investigation.

medicinal plants or herbs which can be used by them after delivery.

Herbalists: Baiga in Chhattisgarh and Vaidus in Maharashtra

The role of Baiga and Vaidu as traditional practitioners of AYUSH systems of health care at village level was important for promotion of herbal medicines. Their knowledge was gained from their previous generations and the source could be traced from their genealogy in Chhattisgarh. These local health care providers practice in their specialized fields and people have faith in them. They are the only available health care providers in the absence of ANMs and doctors of Allopathy or AYUSH. They bring fresh herbal material from backyard or nearby forest in the form of roots, leaves, flowers, tubers or bark and prepare dispensable medicine.

Baigas in Chhattisgarh

Thirty six Baigas from 16 villages of 2 blocks were interviewed. 18 Baigas each from 2 blocks were covered. 24 Baigas belonged to 4 tribal groups namely Gonds, Bhaina, Oraon and Kanwar and 12 were non-tribals. Their age ranged from 40 to 80 years. Interview revealed that they treat large number of patients for piles, distention of abdomen, jaundice, malaria, fever, kidney stones, arthritis, paralysis, all types of pain, e.g. headache, abdominal pain, cancer, diarrhoea, skin problems, menstrual problems, white discharge, epilepsy, snake and scorpion bites and some other minor ailments. They informed about use of approximately 37-40 medicinal plants (which they named and documented) available in the nearby forest for treating the patients. The parts of the plants used by them are given in Table 4.4.

In Chhattisgarh Baiga are using nearly 200 herbs for treatment. In Maharashtra tribal areas under AUK programme 276 Vaidus are trained for processing herbs into medicine in dispensable forms. They were taught to prepare *Bala Teil* for baby's body massage, *Shatavari Kalp* for underweight children and for lactating mothers, *Gandharva Haritaki* as laxative and *Kutajghanvati* for worm infestation in children. For sustainability of this activity trainers were trained in each of the 9 taluks and utensils for processing the herbs were also provided.

Table 4.4: Parts of plants used by Baiga for treatment in Chhattisgarh

Sl. No.	Plant Part	Pendra block		Marwahi block	
		Frequency	%	Frequency	%
1.	Bark	55	34.16	20	17.6
2.	Flower	2	1.24	5	4.4
3.	Fruit	2	1.2	36	31.85
4.	Gum	1	0.62	—	—
5.	Node	1	0.62	—	—
6.	Rhizome	2	1.24	—	—
7.	Root	54	33.54	33	29.2
8.	Seed	6	2.48	—	—
9.	Stem	5	3.1	2	1.76
10.	Tuber	15	9.31	4	3.53
11.	Leaf	5	3.1	10	8.84
12.	Other	13	8.07	3	2.65
	Total	161	100	113	100

Source: Research Team's Field Investigation.

Table 4.5: Ailments treated by Baigas of Chhattisgarh and Vaidu from Maharashtra

Sl. No.	Name of Ailments	Chhattisgarh		Maharashtra
		No. of Herbs used	Products/ forms	Herbs
1.	Fever	8	5	6
2.	Malaria	19	11	—
3.	Jaundice	20	8	9
4.	Bone setting	03	04	1
5.	Piles	19	10	3
6.	Arthritis	15	07	5
7.	Cough and cold	10	04	—
8.	Stomach pain	06	06	5
9.	Skin Disease	06	04	—
10.	Toothache	01	01	4
11.	Headache	02	02	1
12.	Dhaat	06	04	—
13.	T.B.	11	04	—
14.	Gynaec Problems	41	16	11
15.	Cancer	01	01	—
16.	Paralysis	14	04	1
17.	Filaria	01	01	—
18.	Snake/Scorpion Bite	03	03	10
19.	Diarrhaea	01	01	13
20.	Renal Calculi	07	04	10
21.	Worm Infestation	—	—	4
22.	Avoid Miscarriage	—	—	3
23.	For conception	—	—	5
24.	To increase weight	—	—	4
25.	Lactation + Recovery after delivery	06	03	7

Source: Research Team's Field Investigation.

The medicines are processed by them, following spiritual rituals. For getting optimum results from their herbal medicines, they advice *Parhej* (food restrictions), i.e. avoiding sour and spicy food because they think that medicines do not act if food restrictions are not followed. They informed that forest depletion had reduced the availability of good quality medicinal plants. They have to walk a distance up to 10 km in search of the required herbs. They informed that they were treating village people since the time of their ancestors and did not ask for any money. Voluntarily people offered coconut, grains, incense sticks, chicken or liquor. They examined patients based on their knowledge about *Naadi* (Pulse) in the morning and evening only to diagnose the health problem. Without *Naadi* examination they did not treat a patient. Most of them wanted further training to process the medicinal plants.

Baiga/Herbalist from Madhya Pradesh

Sixteen villages under Sagar and Kesli blocks were studied. Ten herbalists from these sixteen villages were interviewed. The herbalists treat both men and women suffering from weakness, body ache, broken bones etc. They prefer using fresh herbs for treatment as they are more effective. The herbalists are also involved in ANC and PNC care and carry out difficult or complicated deliveries. The herbalists give medicines to improve lactation and can help to expedite labour in difficult cases. They also give medicines for menstrual problems and leucorrhoea. The herbalists have remedies for illnesses such as chronic fever, stomach ache, body ache and give medicines for digestive problems. Along with humans, some herbalists also treat animals. They deal with veterinary problems and carry out complicated deliveries of domestic cattle.

Baiga from Manjhagava village treats physical weakness, body aches and does bone setting. He is very popular. People from far off places come to call him. According to him, "to promote Ayurved more awareness efforts are needed. People who can recognize medicinal plants can do this work better. Many Baigas do not use medicines in proper doses. To prepare medicines Baigas need training in processing of medicinal plants and dispensing the medicines. This should be done at village level by using fresh plants."

In Maharashtra, herbalists who are called Vaidus are the main providers of health care in tribal areas. In Etapalli block in Gadchiroli district which is adjacent to Bastar in Chhattisgarh, having good forest cover, four tribal vaidus reported problems of getting medicinal herbs from the forest due to encroachment of forest land for agriculture. They use atleast 42 varieties of herbs and trees for day-to-day use as medicine. They have now planted some herbs near their houses.

A Thakar tribal vaidu trainer from Karjat block in Raigad district near Mumbai could enumerate 353 varieties of medicinal herbs and plants and knowledge about the parts such as root, leaves, flowers, skin, fruits of these plants which are used for their medicinal properties. The author was a witness to a discussion among three vaidus in Nashik tribal region who listed orally about 600 varieties of medicinal herbs and plants in their area and their geographical locations. At an annual fair at a temple in Ahmednagar district, the vaidus bring medicinal herbs for sale at the Fair market around the temple. At Amarkantak, where Narmada river originates, there are several Baiga treating the patients and selling herbs.

In the forest area of Bilaspur district in Chhattisgarh, Medicinal Plant Board has erected a herbal clinic-*cum*-sale depot managed by Baigas. At Arogya Mela organized under the auspices of Department of AYUSH, Government of India, at Raipur there were more than 1000 Baigas present.

It is thus quite clear that these herbalists who are a part of the local kinship community are rendering useful services to the people at affordable cost mostly paid in kind. They could be trained to process the herbal material into medicine which could have a better shelf life and improve their economic status. They could also be oriented to the great tradition knowledge to upscale the symptomatic treatment currently offered by them.

Training Needs of Baigas/Vaidus

Training needs of Baigas were identified through their expressions. The herbalists said that many of them did not have the knowledge about the right quantities of herbs to be used and mixed, while making a medicine. Hence, there should be proper training given to herbalists on the processing and preparation of herbal medicines.

Baiga Recommendations from Chhattisgarh

- They do not want their knowledge to disappear gradually.
- To expand their traditional knowledge, they want frequent training from Ayurved doctors.
- Training for identification and processing of medicinal plants to prepare medicines is needed and it should be near their village.
- Training of Baigas on AYUSH lines and incorporating their services in primary health care given through Ayurved dispensaries is the need of Chhattisgarh herbal state.
- Every panchayat should have a land reserved for growing medicinal plants and Baigas of the village should be trained and given the responsibility to maintain and monitor the growth of these plants.
- Monthly village level meetings to disseminate the traditional knowledge of Baigas to the people.
- Baigas should have AYUSH medicines in their kit for dispensing.
- Educated youths of the village should be trained in AYUSH and encouraged to cultivate medicinal plants on mass scale.
- Specialist Baigas should receive more attention for training and improvement of their skills. Their services during birthing process are important.
- Directory and documentation of their knowledge is essential.

Baiga's Opinions

- According to them, Ayurved needs to be promoted by creating awareness among the people. Unless the people are aware about it, it would not get the standing it deserves.
- Locals who can recognize the herbs or have knowledge about the herbs can be useful in creating awareness in the community for promotion of Ayurved.
- Need for update about knowledge of herbs and processing was expressed.

People's Sector has given an important message that people have been managing their health conditions by themselves for thousands of years and still continue to do so in regard to common ailments. Over the years, with observation, experience, they have acquired and transmitted knowledge about the interaction of health, herbs, plants, animals, minerals etc., what in anthropology is understood as a universal Man-Environment relationship. Some amongst the people due to their closer interaction with the forests, such as shepherds, cowherds etc. acquired more knowledge and used it to help others in distress. The elderly and experienced women as family midwives also developed professional skill about mother and child health. It would, therefore, be wise to continue to use their clinical acumen and home based or local prescriptions and available drugs to mitigate the health problems of people. Their knowledge could be up-scaled with the conceptual knowledge from classical texts to develop their capacities in analyzing cause-effect relationships. The diagnostic capabilities and identification of risk factors to use the referral services with the knowledge and skills from modern science could be developed.

The attempts to throttle the traditional services offered by *dai* and herbalists would eliminate the knowledge and experience of lay people in solving minor health issues in the spirit of community self-help. The concerns expressed by lay people, *dais* and local healers need to be addressed sympathetically in the interests of the people. The PRI, CBOs, SHGs, youth groups need to be empowered by the use of non-formal education to continue the spirit of co-operative self-help.

The health care delivery employees who are accountable to upward hierarchical bureaucracy by providing dubious statistics in top down formats can never provide solutions to the health problems of the people. People sector is sustainable and need to be empowered with knowledge and with authority to plan and monitor health care delivery of the public sector.

5
PUBLIC SECTOR
Health Care Delivery

Introduction

Before Independence in August 1947, the public sector was practically non-existent in rural India. The Bhore Committee Report in 1946 recommended the structure and organization of health care in rural areas. However, the actual functioning of government sector of health care began with the Community Development Programme initiated on October 2, 1952 in limited Blocks. Gradually, it spread all over the country as Primary Health Centres and Sub-centres. The Ayurvedic and Unani Health Centres more often mentioned as Ayurvedic and Unani dispensaries were subsequently established in the States.

It appears, the first Government Ayurved College in India was established at Tiruvananthapuram in 1889 followed by Dayanand Ayurved non-government college in 1898 at Jallandhar, and Lalit Hari State Ayurvedic College, Pilibhit in 1899, as a Government Institution. The two exclusive Unani colleges in government sector were established in 1902 in Lucknow and in 1904 at Allahabad. Before 1947, there were 26 Ayurved and 16 Unani colleges in India. Obviously, these colleges had affiliated hospitals for training. It could be surmised that the princely States during British rule had more Ayurved or Unani dispensaries than the Presidencies governed directly by the British. It was reported that a proposal to start an Ayurved college in Bombay (now Mumbai) by British government was declined by Ayurved leaders with an argument that Ayurved was best learnt as *Guru-Shishya* tradition (*Parampara*). There upon Grant Medical College was established in Bombay (Personal communication from Dr. C.G. Pandit).

The government sector in health after Independence actively started with Family Planning Programme to control population growth as major national programme which after the election disaster was rechristened as Family Welfare Programme. Mother and Child Health, Reproductive Child Health were brought in focus in the health sector as also under Social Welfare Programme. Anganwadi programme was initiated in 1975 to prevent infant and child mortality and promote mother and child health (ICDS).

As a result of these efforts, primary health centres and Ayurvedic health centres, and Ayurvedic-Unani dispensaries became the first ever therapeutic centres. The sub-centres under primary health centres have been manned by Auxiliary-Nurse-Midwife (ANM), going to the homes of people to provide ANC care, immunization and make available allopathic medicine for common ailments.

The government sector functions through line departments such as Health and Family Welfare which oversees all systems of medicine. Recently non-allopathic systems have been clubbed together as Indian systems of Medicine and Homoeopathy, now AYUSH as acronym. India has two national health policies having no co-ordination or networking with each other. While operationalising national health and disease control programmes, personnel from all plural systems of medicine in India have to work together under the supervision of allopathic district and State level authorities. One retired Director of health services of undivided Madhya Pradesh (which included Chhattisgarh) told me that the allopathic and ayurvedic doctors were equally good or bad when it came to their participation in the national programmes. After the disbanding of National Malaria Eradication Programme, the malaria workers were absorbed in the PHC set-up as Multipurpose Workers (MPW). After the withdrawal of vertical leprosy control programme, the leprosy technicians or leprosy para-medical workers and non-medical supervisors have been absorbed in the PHC system. Recently, under NRHM, a new category of village volunteer, ASHA (acronym for Accredited Social Health Activist) has been added on task based payment basis as incentive. Earlier, community health volunteer (CHV) or Health guide were appointed. In tribal belt in Maharashtra, Pada (hamlet) workers were appointed to monitor and refer health related issues.

As a result, in rural India we have two categories of health personnel. The doctors, MPWs and ANMs are regular employees in the government system. The Anganwadi workers and ASHA are reporting to the government system, but are paid honorarium, not regular salaries as employees. In traditional culture systems, the *dai* and herbalist (Vaidu, Baiga etc.) have been providing health services to the people, receiving consideration from the people on voluntary basis in cash or kind or a mix of the two.

The organization of AYUSH health care delivery system from state to village level was studied in the four States along with the infrastructure available to deliver the services. AYUSH health institutions were visited at State, district, block and village levels, meetings organized and discussions held with the health functionaries.

AYUSH Medical Education

There are 116 AYUSH undergraduate medical colleges in Maharashtra, the largest number in one State in the country. Out of 116 there are 63 Ayurvedic, 48 Homoeopathic and 5 Unani medical colleges. In West Bengal which is considered as home for Homoeopathy, there are only 13 Homoeopathic colleges as compared to Maharashtra. The Director of Ayurved has the only function to supervise these 116 colleges and attached hospitals as he has no public health responsibility. Most of the AYUSH doctors passing out from these colleges in the absence of getting AYUSH institutional attachments go for private practice and most of them practice allopathy or mixed practice. In States like Himachal where there are only three Ayurved colleges, all the doctors passing out get opportunity to work in AYUSH facilities. Actually there is a shortfall of Ayurved doctors in Himachal Pradesh to man the AHCs. There are 25 per cent vacant posts of doctors at the AHC.

It needs to be understood that bed strength and number of hospitals attached to the colleges are not exclusively used for AYUSH facilities. Most of the hospitals particularly in the Private Sector were already existing as allopathic hospitals before AYUSH colleges were started. The medical personnel available in the AYUSH sector are no indicator about the use of AYUSH facilities by the people. The colleges of all systems of medicine are only providing numbers to manage the National Health Care

Table 5.1: AYUSH Medical colleges, hospitals and dispensaries

State	*Total U.G. Colleges*	*Govternment Colleges*	*Pvt. Colleges*	*Ayur.*		*Homeo.*		*Unani*		*AYUSH Hospitals*	*Beds*	*Disp.*
				G	*P*	*G*	*P*	*G*	*P*			
Maharashtra	116	4	112	4	59	—	48	—	5	105	9612	497
Himachal Pradesh	3	1	2	1	1	—	1	—	—	31	647	1136
Madhya Pradesh	42	9	33	7	11	1	19	1	3	50	2731	1623
Chhattisgarh	8	1	7	1	2	—	3	—	1	14	930	1471
Rajasthan	16	3	13	3	4	—	7	—	2	132	1303	3861

Source: AYUSH in India: 2010.

Table 5.2: System-wise Number of AYUSH Colleges and their Admission Capacity as on 1.4.2010

Medical Systems	*No. of U.G. Colleges*	*Admission Capacity*
Ayurved	254	11927
Unani	39	1757
Siddha	7	350
Naturopathy	10	385
Homoeopathy	185	12371
Total	**495**	**26790**

Source: AYUSH in India 2010: 107/115.

programmes or to cope up with the patient load particularly in the growing urban areas. They need not or do not practice the system of medicine in which they are formally trained. Most of them work in the private sector in urban or peri-urban areas.

It is common knowledge that the sheet anchor of health care delivery are the para-medical staff working at the grassroots although many of them do not reside at work place. The vertical disease control programmes were managed by the para-medics such as in leprosy control programme. Even now while the leprosy vertical programme has been merged in the integrated PHC system, case detection and drug delivery is done by ex-leprosy technicians, now with the PHC. The PHC doctor is not usually involved in leprosy control. This has resulted in the expressed concerns about incidence of leprosy and late reporting of cases with grade deformity. This scenario of leprosy has been validated in the midterm evaluation of NLEP in India during November 2014 undertaken by WHO.

Actually in rural areas, the health workers entering the houses of the people are ANM, Anganwadi worker and now ASHA. The doctors visit if summoned for emergencies and may charge visit fee. Instead of hundreds of Medical Colleges in the country producing the doctors who are trained to treat disease conditions in a symptomatic mode, it is necessary to have training institutes in large number for public health nursing with knowledge of allopathy and AYUSH systems and their respective strengths about preventive, promotive and curative aspects of health.

Shailaja Chandra has emphasized the need for paramedical supporting staff for ASU Colleges, ASU pharmacists, *Panchkarma* and *Ksharsutra* technicians, laboratory technicians, nursing staff, ward boys and librarians which are basic requirements for accreditation of colleges.

Table 5.3: Number of Institutes imparting Para-medical education and their Admission Capacity in India as on 1.4.2010

Ownership	*Ayurved*		*Unani*		*Siddha*		*Homoeopathy*		*Total*	
	No.	*Adm. Cap*	*No.*	*Adm. Cap*	*No.*	*Adm. Cap*	*No.*	*Adm. Cap*	*No.*	*Adm. Cap*
Government	23	790	6	40	2	15	12	255	35	1280
Local Body	1	50	1	20	0	0	0	0	2	70
Private	31	235	25	0	0	0	25	0	31	1235
Total	55	1075	32	60	2	15	37	255	68	2585

Source: AYUSH in India 2010: 118.

Para-medical training in AYUSH refers to diploma/certificate courses as ayurvedic compounder, pharmacist and Mahila health worker.

In Madhya Pradesh, there are 10 Government institutes (7 for compounder and 3 for Mahila health worker) offering one year certificate course. In Chhattisgarh there are 3 Government institutes offering one year course, one each for compounder, *Panchkarma* assistant and *mahila* health worker. In Himachal Pradesh there is one Government centre for 2-year training as Ayurvedic pharmacist. In Rajasthan, there are 4 Government and 25 Non-Government centres offering 3-year diploma course as Ayurvedic compounder/Nurse training.

AYUSH Organisation: AYUSH Health Institutions and Manpower

Himachal Pradesh

In Himachal Pradesh AYUSH department has a separate vertical and parallel system of health care institutions. The health institutional network of Department of AYUSH in the state is well planned and has expanded over several years. Currently there is a well established network of AYUSH health institutions and manpower from districts to AHC/village level.

Important facts are—

- There are 1136 Ayurved Health Centres (AHCs), and 450 PHCs in the state. Both are headed by qualified medical officers.
- The expansion of number of AHCs has taken place not on the basis of population as for PHC, but on the demands from the people and electoral constituencies. Population catered by each AHC varies as per the location. In some areas the AHCs are located at a very short distance from each other and in the vicinity of PHC or SC.
- There is co-location of Homoeopathy and Ayurved at district hospitals. All the 14 district AYUSH (Ayurved) hospitals in the state have Homoeopathic dispensaries.
- There are Sub-divisional Ayurved Health Centres between district and peripheral AHC levels in each district headed by Sub-Divisional AYUSH Medical Officers (SDAMOs) for better monitoring of AHCs. Sub-Divisional Ayurved Medical Officers who besides supervising functioning of AHCs and AYUSH manpower in their regions, also coordinate with District Ayurved Officers.

AYUSH Manpower Salient Features

- Health and Ayurved Minister for Himachal during BJP rule was himself an Ayurved physician.
- There is Directorate of AYUSH at Shimla headed by Director who is from the Civil Services.
- At Directorate, there is one post of Additional Director, 2 Assistant Directors, 1 OSD (HQRS) and administrative staff.
- The Directorate controls Government Ayurved Pharmacies, Ayurved College, Herbal Gardens, Pharmaceutical chemists and District Ayurved Officers (DAOs).
- There are 12 District Ayurved Officers (DAOs) for AYUSH in the state.
- There are 2-3 Sub-Divisional Ayurved Medical Officers (SDAMOs) in each district and Ayurved Medical Officers (AMOs) under each DAO who monitor Ayurvedic Health Centres and AYUSH manpower in their sub-divisions.
- AYUSH health care in the districts is imparted through 1136 AHCs, each manned by AMO and paramedical staff like Midwife and pharmacist and one attendant.

- SDAMOs supervise and monitor AYUSH Health Centres, Unani Health Centres and Amchi Clinics.
- There is a huge backlog between sanctioned and functioning personnel for the posts of AMOs, Ayurvedic pharmacists and midwives, about 25 per cent posts remaining vacant.

In the study district Hamirpur of Himachal Pradesh, there are 74 AHC out of total 1136 in the State and 3 Ayurvedic hospitals out of 25 in the State. In the district, one AHC was opened in the year 1952 which gradually rose to 74 in 2007. At the State level, 230 AMO post are vacant out of sanctioned 1148 as on 31 March, 2009. Similarly, 658 pharmacist out of 1174, 36 ANM out of 190, *Dai* 381 out of 894 and 20 out of 38 laboratory technician posts are vacant. In Hamirpur district. 18 Pharmacist out of 73 posts are vacant and 4 out of 6 staff nurses, 9 out of 56 trained *dai* are yet to be appointed as on May 2009.

The AMO have contributed to the implementation of National Programmes as under:

Table 5.4: Annual National Programmes Report for the Year 2008-09 of District Hamirpur (Himachal Pradesh)

Sl. No.	*National Programmes*	*Sub-Divisions of Hamirpur District*			*Total*
		Sub-Division Hamirpur	*Sub-Division Nadaun*	*Sub-Division Barsar*	
1.	NSV cases	3	3	1	**7**
2.	Condoms	1640	1210	5640	**8490**
3.	Iron Tablets	39400	850	2900	**43150**
4.	D.O.T. Cases	55	59	53	**167**
5.	D.P.T. Vaccine	803	237	181	**1221**
6.	B.C.G. Vaccine	248	5	31	**284**
7.	Hepatitis-B Vaccine	347	196	147	**690**
8.	Lapro. Sterilization	76	35	18	**129**
9.	Contraceptive Pills	539	220	186	**945**
10.	Vitamin "A" Doses	473	55	169	**697**
11.	O.P.V. Drops	479	580	181	**1240**
12.	T.T. to Pregnant Mothers	375	106	65	**544**
13.	Measles Vaccine	268	50	61	**379**
14.	Total School Covered	254	83	54	**391**
15.	Total Children Examined	12929	5783	3270	**21982**

Source: State Government Report.

Annual *Kshar Sutra* Activity Report for the Year 2008-09 of Sub-Division of Hamirpur District (Himachal Pradesh)

(a) Fistula in Ano: 70 Cases
(b) Hemorrhoids: 92 Cases

Annual *Panchkarma* Activity Report for the Year 2008-09 of Sub-Division of Hamirpur District (Himachal Pradesh)

(a) New Patients: 118
(b) Old Patients: 1165

Total Patients: 1283

Table 5.5: Annual Patient Treated Report for the Year 2008-09 of Sub-Divisions of District Hamirpur (Himachal Pradesh)

Sl. No.	*Sub Divisions of Hamirpur District*	*Outdoor Patients*	*Indoor Patients*	*Total Patients*
1.	Sub-Division Hamirpur	206163	618	206781
2.	Sub-Division Nadaun	67701	Nil	67701
3.	Sub-Division Barsar	68989	Nil	68989
	Total	**342853**	**618**	**343471**

Source: State Government Report.

AYUSH Health Information Management System

In Himachal Pradesh there was a systematic documentation of data regarding the different categories of patients treated in AHCs and was seen to be very well documented every month including the medicines dispensed as shown in Table 5.6.

It was observed from district and state level records that large number of patients are treated in AHCs. AHCs were seen and reported to be more crowded than PHCs. There was no awareness and recognition about role and share of AYUSH systems in state health care and participation of AYUSH doctors in national health programmes in the State level health statistics report published by State Department of Health and Family Welfare. There was absence of computerized system of data analysis and a system of MIS. It was not clear as to how this data gets coordinated at district and state level. AYUSH doctors are working for National Health programmes. "Health at a glance" folder published by Director of

Table 5.6: Details of patients treated by AYUSH systems in Himachal Pradesh, 2008-09

Sl. No.	*Particulars*	*Number of patient treated*	*Details*
1.	Naadi Sansthan	4,74,390	Male patients 18,37,384
2.	Pachan Sansthan	6,99,398	Female patients 21,57,428
3.	Rakta Pravah	3,07,392	Children 13,05,896
4.	Shwas Sansthan	7,20,269	
5.	Mutravah Sansthan	7,87,198	**Total 53,00,708**
6.	Twacha Rog	3,89,268	New patients 43,29,519
7.	Eye problems	3,26,574	Old patients 9,71,189
8.	Fever	4,24,697	**Total 53,00,708**
9.	Others	11,71,522	
	Total	**53,00,708**	

Source: Directorate of AYUSH.

Table 5.7: Name of Diseases for which patients generally visited the Government Ayurved Hospitals/Dispensaries and number of patients visited during 2010-11 in Himachal Pradesh (AYUSH in India: 2010)

Sl. No	*System*	*Ayurved*	*Unani*	*Homoeopathy*	*Sowa-Rigpa*
1.	Pachan Sansthan	631250	1412	7627	659
2.	Jwar	507045	869	4375	239
3.	Shwas Sansthan	644727	1614	7413	187
4.	Naadi Sansthan	492972	989	4075	540
5.	Rakta Pravah	265850	879	3016	299
6.	Mutravah Sansthan	165638	582	3316	187
7.	Twacha Rog	441394	713	8959	387
8.	Eye, Ear Problems	208298	404	2479	556
9.	Others	741558	1687	14583	438

Source: Directorate of AYUSH.

Health Services, Himachal Pradesh do not include infrastructure and manpower information of AYUSH Department which are providing health care through 1136 AHCs headed each by a AMO, monitored by SDAMO and DAO with their staff. During discussion with the IAS Director of AYUSH in Himachal Pradesh, he said "AYUSH was a younger brother of allopathic system". The Director of health services in Himachal Pradesh did not know anything about *Ksharsutra Chikitsa*. Communication between the Director of Health Services and Director of AYUSH appeared dismal in all the States.

Facilities in Ayurvedic Health Centres of Himachal Pradesh

Himachal Pradesh is perhaps the only State in India that has Ayurvedic Health Centres, more than the PHCs. In fact there are 1136 Ayurvedic Health Centres, around 450 Primary Health Centres, 70 Community Health Centres, 3000 Sub-centres, 16 District Ayurvedic 10 bedded Hospitals, and 2200 bedded district Hospitals. This reveals the popularity and preference of Ayurvedic treatment among the people of Himachal Pradesh. However, AHCs are only dispensaries with OPD facility only, having no other public health function. There has to be some linkage with the sub-centres for meaningful integration.

The researcher personally visited five AHCs and interviewed the Ayurvedic Doctors of the concerned AHC.

A Case Study of Gahaliya A.H.C.

- **Location**: Gahaliya A.H.C. is situated in Gahaliya village, Nadaun block of Hamirpur district.
- **Rooms in the Building**: A.H.C., Gahaliya has only two rooms.
  - Ayurvedic Physicians Consultation room
  - Store-*cum*-Pharmacy room

Doctor, however, uses the open verandah of the AHC, whenever there is rush.

- **Facilities:** Facilities such as electricity, water, toilet, and bathroom are available.
- **Cleanliness:** The AHC was found to be clean.
- **Staff Position:** AHC Gahaliya has only three staff members including the doctor. There is a pharmacist and a midwife.
- **Eradication of Anaemia in Himachal Pradesh (Anaemia Mukta Himachal):** AHC Gahaliya is involved in eradication of anaemia in H.P. Anaemic patients are detected and the data is sent to District Ayurvedic Officer. Infact, the P.H.C.s also send their data to the CMO. The Government of Himachal Pradesh is trying out AYUSH and Allopathic techniques and therapies to eradicate anaemia in Himachal Pradesh. The prevalence of anaemia

is considered high in Himachal Pradesh. A.H.C. Gahaliya is involved in identifying anaemic children, women and men within its vicinity. A day of the week is assigned for this activity. The doctor was seen at an anganwadi in one village testing the villagers for anaemia.

- **Further Scope for AYUSH:** Dr. Hemraj Sharma, the coordinator of AYUSH study for H.P., Dr. B.D. Soni and other Ayurvedic doctors said the Government of H.P. was keen on trying out "*Ksharsutra*" technique to treat piles and fistula. This technique involves surgery of piles using medicated threads. The thread is tied on to piles and automatically the tip dries and falls off after 3 to 4 days. Even use of '*Panchkarma*' in healing certain disorders could be promoted. This is possible at A.H.C.s provided there is:
    - Quality and enough man power;
    - That AYUSH research experts are recruited in A.H.C.s;
    - That the A.H.C. facilities, amenities and space are planned and improved accordingly;
    - That the A.H.C.s are given equivalent status as of P.H.C.s;
    - That there is regularity of AYUSH medicine supply at the A.H.C. level;
    - That there are sub-centres of AYUSH in villages where there are no allopathic sub-centres; and
    - That there is field staff to popularize AYUSH at the grassroots level.
- **Status of Medicine Supply at AHCs:** Interviews with AHC doctors, staff and personal observation of the research team revealed that medicine supply in AHCs was better than PHCs. In AHC Gahaliya following Ayurvedic medicines were seen by the team.
    1. *Avipattikar Churna*
    2. *Haritaki Churna*
    3. *Arjun Churna*
    4. *Triphala Churna*
    5. *Yawani Khandav Churna*
    6. *Vedantak Ras*
    7. *Kapur Ras*
    8. *Vat Kulatak Ras*

9. *Ekangvir Ras*
10. *Madhu yashti Kashay*
11. *Tulsi Adi Kashay*
12. *Maharasnadi Kashay*
13. *Amrutashtak Kashay*
14. *Purnavashtak Kashay*
15. *Pathyadi Kashay*
16. *Rasayan Vati*
17. *Kutdhan Vati*
18. *Khadiradi Vati*
19. *Lavangadi Vati*
20. *Prabhakar Mishrak Vati*

In view of the good work, some furniture pieces at the AHC have been donated by the local community. The PHC sub-centre and Anganwadi happen to be in the same building (barrack). There is informal interaction among the three facilities. Usually, all AHC doctors have private clinics at their residence which function in the evenings.

Madhya Pradesh: Infrastructure for AYUSH in Public Sector

AYUSH in Public Health

In Madhya Pradesh there is AYUSH Directorate headed by Commissioner who is from Civil Services. There are 2 Joint Directors for Ayurved and Homoeopathy and under them are deputy directors for Ayurved, Homoeopathy and Unani systems. Principals of AYUSH medical colleges are directly under Director. Deputy Directors supervise Divisional Ayurveda Officers, District Ayurveda Officers, Superintendants of Ayurveda, Homoeopathy and Unani hospitals, Superintendats of Ayurved and Unani pharmacies, Drug Controller AYUSH and other administrative staff. There is one Deputy Director for non-technical and administrative matters working under Joint Directors.

Mainstreaming of AYUSH under NRHM has not yet been operationalized at the PHC and SC level. The structure of public Ayurvedic dispensaries is inadequate and lack in the availability of basic amenities such as water supply, electricity and telephone connections. AYUSH OPDs have been started in district hospitals at the district level, but these OPDs are situated in the rear portion of the hospitals which have no visibility. The Ayurvedic Doctors at these OPDs are available only on three days a week and there is no awareness among the patients about AYUSH related health-care facilities and treatment options. They also do not know which ailments can be treated better with AYUSH treatment and which ailments would be better treated by allopathic treatment.

In all the PHCs and SCs there are no separate buildings or rooms for AYUSH related treatment and facilities, neither are there AYUSH doctors nor are AYUSH related medicines supplied at the PHCs or SCs. There is no mention of AYUSH in the PHC or SC reporting forms also.

Table 5.8: AYUSH Dispensaries in Madhya Pradesh

AYUSH Dispensaries	*In Madhya Pradesh*			*In Sagar District*
	Rural	*Urban*	*Total*	
Ayurved	1300	61	1427	48
Unani	23	27	50	6
Homoeopathy	82	64	146	2
Total	1471	152	1623	56

Source: Directorate of AYUSH.

There are large number (1623) of Ayurved, Homoeopathic and Unani dispensaries in Madhya Pradesh each having a trained Medical Officer and the Paramedical staff. If compared with the number of PHCs in the State, each having 2 Medical Officers and the Paramedical staff of PHC and sub-centres it can be seen that AYUSH has larger number of trained manpower as doctors and paramedics which is not properly utilized and popularized for various reasons. Following Table 5.9 shows that in Sagar district there are 48 AYUSH dispensaries and AMOs as compared to 28 PHCs. Tables 5.10 and 5.11 also show the health institutions and health manpower available in selected Sagar and Kesali blocks.

I. Status of Primary Health Centres—Infrastructure

Out of 4 PHCs 3 were situated on the outskirts of villages and were difficult for the villagers for easy access to while one was located in the centre of village and was easily accessible. The Primary Health Centre's buildings were new. All the 4 PHCs had

Table 5.9: Total Public Health institutions in Sagar District (Including AYUSH)

Blocks	*CHC*	*PHC*	*SHC*	*Ayurved Dispensary*	*Homoeopathy Dispensary*	*Unani Dispensary*
11	10	28	245	48	6	2

Source: DAO records, Sagar.

Table 5.10: Public Health institutions in Sagar and Kesali blocks

Blocks	*CHC*	*PHC*	*SHC*	*Ayurved Dispensary*	*Homoeopathy Dispensary*	*Unani Dispensary*
Sagar	1	3	30	5	1	2
Kesali	1	2	21	5	0	0
Total	2	5	51	10	1	2

Source: DAO records, Sagar.

Table 5.11: No. of Anganvadis, ASHA and TBA in Sagar and Kesali blocks

	Anganvadi	*ASHA*	*TBA/Dai*
Sagar	236	71	163
Kesali	151	150	160
Total	387	221	323

Source: DAO records, Sagar.

buildings, operation theatre, delivery room, bathrooms, toilets, wards, office room, drug store and OPD with proper compounds and gates. Only 2 PHCs had separate laboratory and dispensing rooms. The buildings status was satisfactory.

Operation theatres available at all the PHCs were used as a common room for the staff to sit in, or used as kitchen by the staff or used as a storeroom for medical equipments and medicines etc.

All PHCs had two to three staff quarters on campus. The quarters were available for nurses, dressers and Medical Officers. In 50 per cent PHCs doctors were available for 3 times a week. Doctors only worked for 3-4 hours on the days they came. On other 3 days they were working at other places. In the absence of doctors people do not get PHC services.

Observations During Study about Sub-centres

In Kesali block Tada and Kevlari Kala sub-centres under Tada PHC and Amoda and Muhali SCs under Sahajpur PHC were observed. At Tada, PHC and SC were both located in the same village. SC building was not used by MPW for providing health care services due to some problems. Kevalari Kala SC was locked and seen to be out of use. It was reported that ANM charges money for medicines. Women from these sub-centres directly go to PHC.

In Sagar block ANM stays in Amoda SC under PHC. Sahajpur. SC is well maintained. The SC has no contact with Ayurved dispensary located just adjustant to it. ANM Amoda informed about drug shortage specially pain killers and supply of very small sized syringes. Drugs were provided close to expiry date. ANM was complaining about large target for preparing blood smears for diagnosis of malaria. MPW was complaining about delay in receiving smear report and thereby delay in treatment of smear positive cases. Muhali SC of Sagar block was giving proper services in all the villages as the ANM was staying in the village.

II. Study of Ayurved Dispensaries

In the study area of Kesali and Sagar block 3 Ayurved dispensaries, namely Amoda and Kevlari Kala in Kesali block and Vamhori Dhudhar in Sagar block were observed as follows:

1. Ayurved Dispensary at Amoda in Kesali Block

Dispensary is located in Government building with one room and verandah. There is no electricity and water supply and only a table, chair and bench is available. Doctor resides in varandah of same building. He works for 3 days in Amoda and for another 3 days goes on duty to another dispensary. Doctor, patients and staff were not seen. Staff consists of doctor, compounder, *dai* and peon. Patients come infrequently for treatment and the medicines are given by *dai* as she stays in the same building. *Dai* does not conduct delivery. Drug supply was adequate, but not utilized as there are few patients. So, the drugs are used in village fairs for free distribution.

Suggestions of Amoda MO: He feels that he feels embarrassed to face the Allopathy doctor. There is no budget for basic facilities like repairs, cleanliness while the neighbouring SC is given Rs. 10,000 for painting. Paramedical staff of dispensary do not work for which they are appointed.

2. Ayurved Dispensary at Kevlari Kala in Kesali Block

This dispensary is located in Panchayat Bhavan on rental basis. Patients come for treatment. Doctor is available for 3 days and on other 3 days he has to go on duty to some other place. The appointed paramedical staff and doctor were not seen in dispensary. Only compounder works. Monthly report of the dispensary shows only number of new and old cases without any diagnosis, age and sex information.

Demand by Medical Officer of Kevalari Kala: Supply of drugs of good quality, injection availability, drug syrup availability, building, proper system of distribution of medicines, and OPD fees. He said awareness among people about importance of Ayurved and Yoga for remaining healthy is necessary.

In comparison to PHCs and SCs, Ayurved dispensaries are having very bad infrastructure facilities. They do not have own buildings, enough furniture, drinking water supply, electricity and absence of any repair work in the last year.

3. Ayurved Dispensary at Vamhori Dhudhar in Sagar Block

Ayurved dispensary in this village was located in Panchayat Bhavan and was not in good condition. The furniture was not adequate and there was no cupboard for keeping medicines to protect them from rats. The floor was mud plastered and full of dust. There was poor maintenance of the premises. There was no electricity and water supply and toilets. There was no place for medical officer to stay and there were no staff quarters. Medical officer had to commute everyday.

For providing proper health care medical officer of the Ayurved dispensary expressed his views as under:

- There should be separate building for Ayurved dispensary.
- Staff quarters to be there.

- Improve quality of drugs as current drug supply is of low quality and not very effective.
- Supply of drugs in smaller packs for easy dispensing.

I visited a Unani dispensary with DAO in Sagar town located in a lane inhabited by poor muslim community. It was clear that DAO had not visited the dispensary earlier as he could not locate it without the directions given by pharmacist at the clinic on mobile phone. There were women and children in the lane as the men folk had already left for work. It appeared the clinic was useful to women and children as it was free and women could access it without observing *purdah*. There was no Unani doctor posted at the clinic.

Based on above mentioned observations about availability of AYUSH facilities in public sector health care following issues have emerged:

- Government Ayurved dispensaries have poor infrastructure to provide proper health services. Attention is necessary from the AYUSH department for improving the infrastructure.
- Practice of utilizing services of AYUSH practitioners and displacing them from their own place of work creates discontinuity of clinical work and leads to lack of people's trust in the health services. AMOs are sent on locum duties as a routine. Non-availability of AMOs for 6 days in a week at the place of his posting creates discontinuity in clinical work.
- Working time of Medical officers and paramedics for full day needs monitoring.
- Lack of dedication and concern by AYUSH staff towards people was observed.
- AYUSH paramedical staff and AMOs have low self esteem and need morale boosting and treatment at par with PHC staff.
- Lack of community awareness about availing AYUSH health care and strengths of AYUSH leads to less access to AYUSH health care facilities.
- Need for quantitative and qualitative MIS system for reporting of the AYUSH work done by staff. Need for adding AYUSH component in PHC MIS is necessary.

Table 5.12: Annual OPD attendance in AYUSH Dispensaries of Sagar District

No.	Annual OPD attendance in AYUSH Dispensaries of Sagar District—2008-09			
	Patients	*Ayurved Dipensaries*	*Unani Dispensaries*	*Homoeopathy Dispensaries*
	New	2,36,035	8,387	31,454
	Old	48,280	11,263	27,657
	Total	2,84,315	19,650	59,111
	Grand Total	2,84,315	19,650	59,111

Source: DAO records, Sagar.

Table 5.13: Disease-wise Annual OPD attendance in AYUSH Dispensaries of Sagar District—2008-09

Sl. No.	*Disease*	*Total No. of Patients (Old+New)*					
		Ayurved D.	*%*	*Unani D.*	*%*	*Homoeopathy D.*	*%*
1.	Cough	37980	9.63	2469	12.56	5326	9.0
	Asthma	11935	3	1079	5.5	3033	5.13
2.	Cold/coryza	25485		1326		—	
	ENT	20604	5.2	947	4.8	3096	5.2
	Tuberculosis	152		56		395	
3.	Diarrhoea and dysentery	30148	7.64	811	4.12	4302	7.27
	Liver disorders	4254		—		574	
	Worms	7946	2	886	4.5	2097	3.5
4.	Piles	6294	1.5	596	3.0	2085	3.5
5.	Fevers + malaria	35413	9.9	1950	9.0	4393	7.2
6.	Measles/ Chicken pox	124		158		520	
7.	Skin disease, leucoderma	27925	7.08	3691	18	6632	11.2
8.	Gynec. problems	21061	5.34	1950	9.92	5025	8.50
	STD	976		—		705	
9.	Vatrog + Neurological	32416	8.2	1580	8	3856	6.52
	Epilepsy	402		—		385	
10.	Diabetes	1079		737		830	
11.	Heart disease	1473		585		611	
12.	Jaundice/anaemia	3339		—		390	
13.	Others	123921	31	829	4.2	9091	15.3
	Total	**394314**		**19650**		**59111**	

Source: DAO records, Sagar.

Following table shows the number of patients treated by Ayurved, Unani and Homoeopathy systems in Madhya Pradesh.

The data from above Table 5.12 shows that large number of patients are taking treatment from Ayurved, Unani and Homoeopathic dispensaries of the Sagar district.

Observations about Public Sector Health Institutions Including AYUSH

From the above observations it was clear that as per policy public sector health institutions were in place in the study area. But the health facilities provided by them were found to be inadequate. The people were not able to derive benefits from the available facilities. In villages where health institutions were not located, ASHA and local health workers provided the services.

Ayurved dispensaries were not being used by people. There were huge shortfalls as regards AYUSH infrastructure facilities and manpower. The Ayurvedic doctors at these OPDs were available only on three days a week and there was no awareness among the patients about availability of AYUSH related health-care facilities and treatment options.

For mainstreaming, all public sector health care units including Ayurved dispensaries will need to be improved in infrastructure and manpower availability. Communication between AYUSH, Primary Health Centres, Sub-Centre health units is very important for mainstreaming. Private doctors do not necessarily give quality treatment, but still people go there because public health services are not available in times of need. Private facilities are available on demand and payment.

Status of Co-location

Mainstreaming of AYUSH under NRHM was not operationalized at the PHC and SC level. Co-location was not seen. In all the PHCs and SCs there was no space for AYUSH related facilities, neither were there AYUSH doctors nor AYUSH drugs. There is no mention of AYUSH in the PHC or SC MIS reporting forms also.

In the newly constructed district hospital, separate Ayurved and Homoeopathy OPD facilities were made available in the backyard of the building with round about access. There is no interaction among the Ayurved dispensaries and PHCS, SCs, ASHA, ANMs and traditional healers. There is no awareness among people about the selection of a particular treatment system useful for their health problems. Although the Ayurved doctors and the employees at PHCs and SCs take each other's help in the implementation of National health programmes and vaccination drives, there is no formal documentation and reporting of the same. This interaction is witnessed only at the administrative level and not formalized at policy level.

For Mainstreaming of AYUSH

1. PHC, SC and AYUSH dispensaries should have basic facilities and have close communication with each other.
2. ASHA, AWW, traditional healers need training about AYUSH so that people can get benefits from them.
3. All health workers should jointly provide health services at village level, so, that people will get good quality and trustworthy health care.

Health Manpower in the Public Sector

Health workers in public sector include all the health workers including medical officers who are working for Government programmes and are paid for them. The staff of Primary Health Centres, Sub-centres, Anganwadis, ASHA, AYUSH health centres are referred as health manpower of public sector. All 16 (100%) villages covered had Anganwadi Workers (AWW) and helpers. 62.5 per cent villages had ASHA, 37.5 per cent villages had ANM and MPW both, while 66.66 per cent villages had ANM and 6.25 per cent villages had Ayurvedic doctors.

Health Manpower of Public Sector at Village Level

As regards availability of local resident health workers, besides Anganwadi workers who were available in all the villages, traditional healers (Baiga/Vaidu) in 87 per cent villages, ASHA in 78.78 per cent villages, TBA/*Dais* in 73.33 per cent and ANMs in 66.66 per cent villages were available as resident health workers. MPWs do not stay in villages of work. 25 per cent villages had private doctors. Private quacks like RMPs or retired compounders treat nearly one fourth population. AYUSH facilities had negligible role in the study area.

Status of health care availability at village level through ANMs:

- In the study area most of the villages did not have a separate building for the SC and the SCs are attached to the Anganwadi buildings.
- The villages that have a proper building and equipments lack in the maintenance of these. In most of the villages only one of the two appointed staff works properly.
- The availability of medicines at SCs is not satisfactory. Most of the time villagers have to visit the PHC for treatment and medicines.
- The ANMs carry out check-ups of the pregnant and lactating women *via* the Anganwadi centre or by calling the women on 'Clinic day' at the SC.
- The ANMs are supposed to live in the village itself, but there is no facility for their accommodation and in many villages the ANM resides outside the village.
- Facilities such as accommodation, some mode of transportation, proper equipments, training to use these equipments, proper buildings, and good stock of medicines should be made available to the ANMs.
- They should also be made aware about the various government schemes and the facilities available under these schemes along with the involvement of the Panchayat.

Anganwadis in Study Area

During the study 25 Anganwadis, 16 from six villages in Sagar Block and nine from eight villages in Kesali Block were studied No mini-Anganwadis were found in the study area. AWWs were interviewed for getting information about their own and community's knowledge, perceptions, awareness and utilization about AYUSH services or traditional Ayurved based health practices and home remedies.

Anganwadi workers are important residential health functionaries at village level as they are in contact with every house of the village through their repeated home visits and yearly household surveys. The Anaganwadi workers are health functionaries who with the help of ANM are responsible for providing health care at village level. Majority of the AWWs were 12th pass and a few of them were either graduates or post-graduates.

According to the AWWs the women in the villages have become aware about their health and consult the AWWs and ANMs regularly for health related concerns. The AWWs along with the ANMs carry out regular check-ups and vaccinations of the pregnant and lactating women.

The AWWs carry out certain programmes for the adolescent girls also. These girls are given training in '*Rangoli*' and '*Mehendi*' making. They are also given informal education on health, hygiene, menstruation and life skills. The AWWs prepare the health grade chart of the children registered at the Anganwadi and provide them with nutritious meals. They provide the necessary facilities to the children with low health grade.

The AWWs informed that earlier they used to get kits of Ayurvedic medicines for treating minor ailments but for the last 3-4 years this has stopped. According to them these medicines were very useful and quite popular and should be provided to them again. They also informed that earlier they used to get kits containing modern medicines for common ailments and contraceptives but now this too has stopped. Now all they get are iron tablets for distribution to women which women in the villages do not take, as most of them say they are allergic to it or suffer from side-effects.

The AWWs used home remedies for common ailments using ingredients that are available in the kitchen or locally available. They provide information about such home remedies and the ingredients to be used among the villagers too. They informed that they were not given any training related to home remedies or ingredients that can be used for common ailments during the training period and would like to get such training. They have developed this knowledge through the traditional practices and information passed on through generations by their elders. The AWWs interviewed did not have proper information about the NRHM scheme.

According to the AWWs who are local community women and who are in contact with most of the village households following views were expressed:

- The women in the villages have become aware about their health and consult the AWWs and ANMs regularly for health related concerns.
- During pregnancy the women who are economically better-off take extra care about their diet and nutritional requirements. The AWWs help the women who are financially less well-off in maintaining a balanced diet too.
- According to the AWWs, during pregnancy the women do not take any extra supplements or herbal medicines, but follow traditional ANC practices. They do not take rest during pregnancy, but continue working regularly till the 6th or 7th month of pregnancy.
- As PNC after delivery the new mothers take traditional body massage for 15-20 days.
- The new born are also given regular oil massage at least for 4-6 months. The new born are exclusively breast-fed for 4-5 months and then given weaning food.

List of documents maintained at all the Anganwadis:

1. Register documenting number of days of informal education at the Anganwadi (3-6 years)
2. Register documenting distribution of nutritious food
3. Register documenting number of children in the age group of 6 months to 3 years registered at the Anganwadi
4. Documentation of Women's Groups
5. Documentation of vaccination drives
6. 'Kishor Balika' training documentation
7. 'Kishor Balika' Club documentation
8. Documentation of number of births
9. Documentation of number of deaths
10. Documentation of number of marriages
11. Documentation of the Anganwadi stock
12. Documentation of the weight of pregnant women, young girls and children registered at the Anganwadi
13. 'Baal Sanjivani' documentation

14. 'Laadli Lakshmi Yojana' documentation
15. 'Mangal Divas' scheme register
16. 'Home-tech' scheme register
17. Daily documentation diary
18. Inspection and monitoring documentation
19. Movable property documentation

Recommendations by Anganwadis

1. The AWWs should be provided with equipments such as blood pressure machine, stethoscope etc. and they should be properly trained in using these equipments.
2. They should be trained about the use and benefits of Ayurvedic medicines and they should in turn train the members of the various women's groups in the same.
3. The workers at the Anganwadis wanted to be trained in AYUSH related health practices and such training should be provided to them.
4. AYUSH related nutritional supplements should be included in the nutritious food supplied at the Anganwadis.

ASHA in Madhya Pradesh

ASHA assists ANMs and AWW in the implementation of various health programmes. Under the "Janani Suraksha Yojana" programme, the ASHAs get a fixed amount of money for taking a pregnant woman to the hospital for institutionalized childbirth. They get paid an amount of Rs. 150 per vaccination they help in carrying out. They do not have much information about NRHM and they have not been given any training regarding Ayurveda or traditional health practices.

Issues identified during study about ASHA and AYUSH:

- ASHAs were not given training regarding AYUSH and showed willingness to have proper training about AYUSH.
- Educational qualifications for appointment of ASHA should be increased as many of them in the study area could not properly read Hindi language books given to them.

- Performance or work based honararium given to ASHA should be in the form of fixed amount of honorarium or as salary.
- ASHA should be included in AYUSH related programmes and health missions.
- Family support to ASHAs as observed during study needs encouragement and acknowledgement by authorities for their indirect contribution in health care of community. It was reported by some ASHAs that their husbands and family members help them by accompanying them during training to look after young children or for commuting with them for receiving honorarium.
- The ASHAs are local community health functionaries appointed under NRHM. They assist the AWWs and ANMs in the implementation of various health schemes at the village level.
- They have not been given any AYUSH related training and do not have much information about the NRHM scheme.
- They use home remedies for common ailments at household level and they have this information from their elders. They have knowledge about common herbs and kitchen ingredients used in herbal preparations. They spread this knowledge among the locals too.
- They advocate the use of traditional practices and home remedies but are somewhat skeptic about certain practices such a working during pregnancy and lifting heavy weights during pregnancy etc. They think that not being extra careful during pregnancy and continuing to work in the regular manner might lead to complications.
- During the survey it was found that in some villages ASHA has not been appointed as the local women could not pass the criteria for ASHA's appointment. Only three out of eight villages in the study area had ASHA appointed in them. The Sarpanch and the Secretary of the Gram-panchyat informed that ASHAs were not appointed in all the villages as the women in these villages could not pass the examination held for the ASHA.

Health-care Options for the People through Public Sector Services

The people have the options of public health-care facilities, private doctors or getting treated by quacks. Majority of the health-care facilities in the rural areas were found to be provided by ASHA, TBA, ANM, private practitioners and quacks. The availability of AYUSH facilities were found to be negligible. 85.45 per cent people were found to be following allopathic treatment options, and even though the condition and availability of AYUSH treatment facility was found to be poor, still 40 per cent of the people showed acceptability and reliance towards AYUSH treatment options. It was found that though the building and structural components of PHCs and SCs were found to be quite adequate in the villages, the medical facilities available there were inadequate, especially in terms of available manpower due to which majority of the people depended on private doctors and quacks for treatment. Even though the private facilities lacked in proper structure and high quality treatment, majority of people opted for private health care because timely care was not available at the PHCs or SCs. It was found that 90 per cent people opted for visiting private doctors as first line of health care. Only 10 per cent people opted to go to District Hospital at Sagar. It was found that one-fourth of the rural population was being treated by unqualified private health care providers.

This gap on the part of PHCs and SCs and Ayurved dispensaries in public sector can be minimized by the mainstreaming of AYUSH in public health and by starting AYUSH related healthcare at PHC and SC levels.

Chhattisgarh

AYUSH Institutions

As in Himachal Pradesh and Madhya Pradesh, AYUSH has a separate vertical and parallel system of health care in the State.

At State level Chhattisgarh is headed by Director of AYUSH who is trained in Ayurved and has 1 Joint Director, 1 Deputy Director, 1 OSD, and Administrative staff in the Directorate Office. AYUSH colleges are managed by a separate Deputy Director, and

Principals. For Drug testing laboratory and research centre there is a Controller, one Deputy Director for Pharmacy, and there are District Ayurved Officers.

In Chhattisgarh there is one Government Medical College hospital, 6 District Ayurved Hospitals (30 bedded each), 634 Ayurved dispensaries, 52 Homoeopathy and 6 Unani dispensaries under AYUSH department. In the year 2006-07, 5.58 lakhs of patients were benefited through 6641 AYUSH health camps.

Health Infrastructure and Available Health Manpower in the Selected Blocks

- In Pendra block there are 5 PHCs, 17 sub-centres, 5 health supervisors, 28 health workers, 360 Mitanins and 120 Aaganwadi workers.
- In Marwahi block there are 3 PHCs, 27 sub-centres, 12 supervisors, 33 health workers, 438 Mitanins, and 218 Aaganwadi workers.

There is absence of basic infrastructure facilities like water supply, electricity, telephone in the 2 PHCs and in Ayurved dispensaries of Pendra block.

The status of basic facilities like electricity, water supply at PHCs in Marwahi block is better but their absence in Ayurved dispensary.

Infrastructure in PHC, SC and AHC under study:

1. Out of 4 PHC, two had water facility and the other two had to draw water from hand pump.
2. Most of SC had no building of their own. ANM residence was used as SC.
3. All the three AHCs had to draw water from hand pump.
4. In Pendra block, both PHC had no separate electrical connection. The electricity was borrowed from nearby houses or directly from the electric pole. In Marwahi block, both PHCs had electrical connection.
5. SCs had no electric connection in both blocks.
6. AHCs had no electric connectivity.
7. All four PHCs had beds which were very unclean. The AHCs had no beds.

8. There was no refrigerator, telephone or vehicle in any health facility centre.
9. All four PHCs had a building of which three were newly constructed.
10. AHC buildings were very old out of which one had rented accommodation.

Recommendations of PHC Allopathic Medical Officers

- PHCs running in sub-centre buildings need urgent attention.
- Vacant posts need to be filled.
- Beds, generators, X-ray machines, vehicles need to be made available.
- Co-location for AYUSH treatments should have separate room.

Recommendations of Ayurved Doctors of Ayurved Health Centres

- Ayurved dispensaries should have Government buildings.
- Doctors want residential quarters near Ayurved dispensary.
- Staff vacancies to be filled.
- Frequent CME programmes to get update on Ayurved research and advances.
- Ayurved drug supply to be provided in small packs for easy dispensing.
- Ayurved to be popularized in villages with the help of posters and slogans.

ANMs

Seven ANMs were interviewed. They have enough medicines, but do not have Sub-centre buildings. People first go to chemist shop and then to ANMs. None of them knew about NRHM and the word AYUSH. They received help from Mitanins, Aaganwadi workers and *Dais* for immunization and national programmes. They expressed desire for training in AYUSH.

ANM Recommendations

- Sub-centre building and residential quarters should be there.
- They should receive training about AYUSH and Ayurvedic drugs.
- At sub-centre, Allopathic and Ayurvedic drugs should be available but should have separate rooms.
- Sub-centre to be equipped with delivery facilities.
- Aaganwadi workers help them in immunization and implementation of national programmes, so, the 12th pass Aaganwadi workers after receiving training should be linked to the concerned sub-centre.

Aaganwadi Workers

Thirty five Aaganwadi centres were visited in 2 blocks out of which 3 were Mini Aaganwadis. In all Aaganwadis ANM keeps certain allopathic medicines like Paracetamol, Septran etc. It was reported in one Aaganwadi that a Home remedies kit used to be supplied to Aaganwadis before 2008. It contained Ayurvedic medicines to treat common ailments like cold, cough, fever, indigestion, vomiting, diarrhoea etc. It contained following medicines:

1. *Tasiladi Churna*—for cough
2. *Khadiradi vati*—for sore throat
3. *Dadimyatusam vati*—for fever, *apach, yaman*
4. *Godanti mixture*–for headache, bodyache
5. *Laghuvishgarbh tail*—for musculoskeletal pain
6. *Avipattikar churna*—for flatulence and acidity
7. *Kutajghan vati*–for diarrhoea, dysentery
8. *Lashunadi vati*—for pain in abdomen
9. *Balchturbhadra*—for children's ailments like diarrhoea, vomiting, cough, cold etc.
10. *Panchsakar churna*—for constipation
11. *Agnisandipan churna*—for vomiting
12. *Rajpravartani vati*—for pain or less flow during menstruation.

The medicines in the kit were from pharmacy department of Jamnagar, Gujarat University and the kit was received from Block level ICDS office. The Aaganwadi worker informed that these medicines were good and were in demand by people as they gave quick relief. For dispensing these medicines they were paid Rs. 200 per kit.

It was observed by our investigators that the unused medicines were not preserved properly and they were spoiled. There was no expiry date on the packs so they are hesitant for dispensing them.

Initiatives of Anganwadi

- "*God-Bharai*" ceremony done by Anganwadi worker for every registered pregnant woman in the 6 month of her pregnancy.
- "*Anna-Prashan*" ceremony of children of 6 month age is conducted by all Anganwadi centres. In this ceremony children eat *Kheer* (porridge) as first weaning food.
- To educate the adolescent girls for reproductive health.
- Water Purification at the village level has also to be done by Anganwadi Worker.
- First Tuesday of every Month "Vaccination" work done by ANM at Anganwadi Centre.
- Health and Nutrition related information given to all the beneficiaries.
- Help in all National Programmes like, Polio Control, Filaria Control etc.

Recommendations of Anganwadi Workers

- The AYUSH kits should be again given to them as people demand and they can also get Rs. 200.
- AYUSH component to be added in their training which is absent at present.
- They need training about Ayurvedic drugs and their use.

Mitanins as Healthcare Providers

Mitanin programme of Chhattisgarh is a unique Community Health Volunteer programme to address the health needs of people at hamlet and village level. Mitanin means a special kind of friend in local tribal tradition. Mitanin means publicly acknowledging bonding of 2 families for 3 generations as friends and the ritual consists of taking oath and exchange of coconuts amongst the relatives from both families. Government has used this local cultural term Mitanin for ASHA. Mitanin is a married woman from local community, not necessarily formally educated (though most are literate) and is selected by village community through Gram-sabha and endorsed by panchayats. There is a set of processes for her selection which is facilitated through social mobilization activities like Kalajathas.

The Mitanin programme is a part of the health system reforms and was started during Sector Investment Programme of GOI. The programme does not focus only on demand generation and community health aspects in isolation, but is integrated with a range of health sector reforms that aim to strengthen the public health system. The funding is performance based and grants are released quarterly after attainment of milestones set for Mitanins and as well as for public health system to make it more functional. Mitanin programme has been linked to TBA training, coordination of MPWs, improved community based disease surveillance approaches, strengthening of referral services, local Health Information Management data base System (HIMS) and strengthening panchayat role and public system accountability. At district level district RCH society and district coordination committee provides leadership. The programme is monitored by State Health Resource Centre and implemented through different NGOs in the state.

The role of Mitanin is like ASHA. She facilitates access to health services, gives first aid and treatment for common ailments, helps prompt referrals, facilitates community based disease prevention activities, imparts health education to women and helps to empower them.

Locally Mitanins are supported by women's health committee, health and ICDS workers. For every 20 Mitanins there is one Block Resource Person (BRP). At block level there is a team of 20 BRPs coordinated by a team of 3 District Resource Persons –DRPs (1 Government and 2 volunteers). In Marwahi block there are 66 Gram panchayats, 2 DRPs, 20 BRPs or block trainers or 'Preraks' and 438 Mitanins and the programme is implemented by the NGO

"Bharat Gyan Vigyan Samiti". In Pendra block there are 33 Gram panchayats, 2 DRPs, 20 BRPs and 360 Mitanins and is implemented by NGO "Chatra Evam Samaj Kalyan Shikshan Prashikshan Samiti".

The training of Mitanin is organized systematically. She receives 12 days camp based and 30 days on the job training. Mitanins receive continuous training through Block Resource Persons-BRPs. The training in home remedies, the supply of drugs through BRPs and the booklet *'Jadi Buti Lae Karo Ilaj'* (Herbs for treatment) helps these women to serve the community. Another booklet 'Jug Jug Jiye Nanheman'(About MCH & RCH) given to them after training helps them to care for pregnant, lactating women and children. They can guide women about baby bath, lactation, massage etc. Every month there is a village meeting of all the Mitanins, BRP with Sarpanch, Gramsevak and villagers where health matters, sanitation etc. are discussed for getting help from Gram Panchayat. Mitanin's kit contains Allopathic medicines like Paracetamol for pain relief and fever, Albendazole for worms, furazolidone as anti-diarrhoeal, Cotrimaxozole, chloroquine, iron and folic acid tabs, first aid material for injuries, pregnancy test kit, contraceptives and weighing machine etc. In March 2009 meeting it was decided that 12th pass Mitanins can go for ANM training.

List of Medicines in the Kit

1. Paracetamol tablet
2. Co-trimoxazole tablet
3. Aluminimum Hydroxide-Magnesium Hydroxide and Methylpolysiloxane tablet
4. Ferus Sulphate with Folic Acid tablet
5. Albendazole tablet
6. Furazolidone tablet
7. Chloroquine tab
8. Gama Benzene Application
9. Gentian Violet solution
10. Rancotrim
11. Glass slide
12. Cotton
13. Spirit

14. Bandage
15. Weighing Machine for Children (Infantometer)
16. Needle (Lancet)
17. Nischay Pregnancy test kit
18. Mala-N tablet
19. Nirodh Condoms

Total Mitanins covered in the 2 blocks were 94. The number of Mitanins per village varied from 2 to 10. 94 per cent Mitanins were from 21 to 45 age group and except 3 per cent all were literate, (mostly from primary to middle school level). Mitanins were motivated to undertake the work by ANMs, village panchayats and other health workers. However, 90 per cent Mitanins in Marwahi block and 23 per cent in Pendra block were self-motivated.

Table 5.14: Training of Mitanin for Mainstreaming of AYUSH

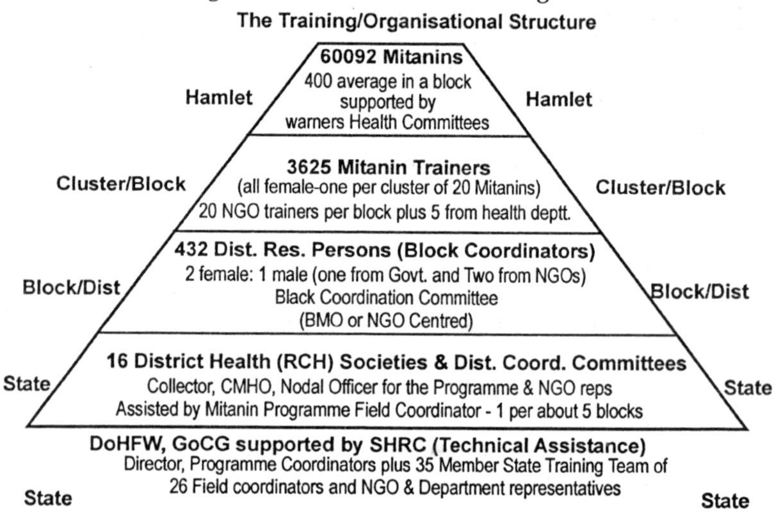

Training of 60,092 Mitanin by inclusion of AYUSH module *"Jadi buti lae karo ilaj"* as propagation and utilization of Herbal combinations for common ailments by Mitanins.

Jadi Buti Lae Karo Ilaj: The AYUSH Training module:

- Ayurvedic concepts on healthy living: The *Swasthavritha.*

- Common diseases and herbal remedies to address them.
- Preservation of herbs and preparation of herbal combinations.
- Do's and don't in traditional/rural health practices.
- Glossary of herbs with pictures and local names.
- There are 15 training booklets for Mitanins dealing with neonate, children and woman's health care, village sanitation, home remedies, disease control about malaria, TB, Leprosy, HIV and AIDS, cataract and insurance schemes. In addition, there is village health register and Mitanin diary.

Mitanin Recommendations about AYUSH

- First aid kit of Mitanins should contain allopathic and AYUSH medicines and have regular supply from district Ayurved office.
- They should receive training about the use of AYUSH and allopathic drugs.
- Medicine supply for children especially syrups should be more.
- ANMs do not allow them to take cases to hospital for delivery and when they go to hospital do not treat them properly. Government should look in the matter.
- Training demand from most of the Mitanins about training in AYUSH and Home Remedies.
- The booklet *"Jadi Buti Lae Karo Ilaj"* is very useful.
- More training related to the use of home remedies with available medicinal plants in the neighbourhood.
- Identification of medicinal plants and their names.
- There should be posters, brochures about AYUSH available to her for explaining to community people.
- Mitanin should be linked to Ayurved dispensaries. Appointment of Mitanins should be formalized by cultural community rituals.
- There should be exposure visits to AYUSH institutions.
- Good work of Mitanins should be acknowledged and they should get cash incentives for that.
- Roles and responsibilities of Mitanins to be clearly sorted out.

- Mobilizing the potentials of 60,000 Mitanins to provide health services in hamlets and villages is a challenging task in Chhattisgarh.

AHC, Kotami, Pendra Block: Case Study

AHC has three rooms, one for the doctor, one for pharmacy and third for other staff. AHC has a doctor, an ANM, compounder and sweeper. There is electrical connection, but water has to be drawn from a hand pump. The OPD is of the order of 600-700 patients per month for treatment of fever, cough-cold, dysentery, respiratory problems, skin, gynec. complaints, ENT, piles, diabetes, injuries etc. Patients ask for injections for quick relief. However, if they are given Ayurvedic drugs in attractive packing they are happy. According to the doctor, the supplies are made in big containers, which have to be dispensed in small packing to patients. The other issue is that the Ayurvedic drugs have to be taken in the medium of honey, milk or ginger juice at home which is cumbersome as compared to allopathic tablets or capsules. Kotmi AHC is popular in the area as the government staff in the Kotmi PHC jurisdiction use AHC facility. The doctor also had his private clinic at his residence.

Mainstreaming: Innovative Approaches

- An innovative scheme "Ayurveda Gram" conceptualized and initiated: this aims to promote AYUSH based lifestyle and health education. 121 villages covered so far successfully.
- AYUSHDEEP Samiti (improved Rogi Kalyan Samiti in line with allopathic facilities) being established for AYUSH facilities may be the first state to initiate this. Special grants being allocated under European Union-Chhattisgarh State Partnership programme.
- 65000 Mitanins (ASHAs) are trained for home based herbal remedies. A manual *"Jadi Buti lae karo ilaj"* developed for this purpose.
- Training of Anganwadi Workers and ANMs on AYUSH based maternal care.

- 325 AYUSH Doctors appointed on contract basis in allopathic health facilities of tribal areas to cater to the shortage of MBBS doctors.
- Recruitment of 399 AYUSH Physicians through PSC is in final stage.
- 198 Pharmacists/Compounder appointed.
- Appointment of contractual Teaching Staff in Ayurveda college.
- AYUSH ANMs under training.

AYUSH Health Services in Primary Health Network

- Co-location of 85 AYUSH dispensaries in PHC/CHC
- 399 Posts of AYUSH Doctors created in PHC and CHC
- 15 AYUSH wings in District Hospitals
- 22 Specialized therapy centres in CHC
- 24 AYUSH specialty clinics in CHC/PHC

Maharashtra

In Maharashtra there is Director AYUSH (Ayurved) at State level. Director AYUSH (Ayurveda) controls State AYUSH colleges and the attached hospitals. There is Deputy Director Homoeopathy and 3 Regional Assistant Directors placed at Pune, Nagpur and Nanded. Director has no public health function because at district and block levels, AYUSH is integrated with general health care system delivered through PHCs, and Ayurveda dispensaries are under DHO. At each DHO office there is one Ayurveda Extension officer for supervising Ayurved dispensaries and also to help the work of Regional Assistant Director. There is no District level AYUSH Health Officer equivalent to DHO. Each Regional Assistant Director supervises government and aided AYUSH medical colleges and their attached hospitals in their regions. With the help of extension officers placed in DHO Office Assistant Directors also monitor the Ayurvedic dispensaries of the state without having any powers. So, Ayurved dispensaries are under dual control of DHO as well as Assistant Director.

In Maharashtra, there is a policy of integration of AYUSH in health care delivery at PHC level. There is co-location at PHC level as BAMS doctors are posted in PHCs. But there is a mismatch between supply and availability of Ayurved drug kits and posting BAMS doctors at PHCs. BAMS doctors cannot practice Ayurved in the absence of supply of Ayurved medicines. Only 25 per cent PHC are supplied with the Ayurved drug kits and this supply does not match with PHCs having Ayurved doctors. So, despite having physical co-location of doctors, AYUSH systems are not practiced. The transfer policy of frequent transfers of the doctors every 2-3 years leads to continuation of this problem of mismatch.

Non-availability of Ayurved drug kits uniformly in all PHCs and non-availability of BAMS doctors in all the PHCs are the major gaps for benefits of co-location and integration in Maharashtra. This is due to absence of powers at State level to AYUSH authorities to monitor AYUSH care in public health delivery system. On the ground, BAMS doctors are found in tribal PHCs where MBBS doctors are not available. These numbers get projected as AYUSH manpower at the State level commensurate with the requirements of mainstreaming under NRHM.

National Scenario

Infrastructure

In general in all the four States there was poor State of AYUSH buildings, inadequate furniture, lack of electricity and water supply in dispensaries, poor instrumentation and lack of vehicles. Even the sub-centres of PHCs in Himachal Pradesh were better maintained than AHCs due to provision of maintenance grants to SCs. The poor AYUSH infrastructure was reported to be due to scarcity of funds and lack of importance given to AYUSH health care at state policy level. There was no vehicle availability to DAOs for monitoring the working of AYUSH dispensaries. Hired transport was not considered as a functional solution. Ayurvedic dispensaries were hardly visited by district authorities resulting in widespread allopathy practice by AYUSH doctors and less attention to promote AYUSH. As a result doubts are expressed about the statistics of OPD attendance submitted to DAO where Ayurvedic and Unani dispensaries are located in the periphery.

AYUSH doctors were most vocal about their marginalized status in health system due to poor infrastructure and lack of recognition of AYUSH systems by Allopathy professionals due to their ignorance about the strengths of AYUSH.

In Himachal Pradesh, Madhya Pradesh and Chhattisgarh States there are approximately 70 AYUSH health centres per district and are supervised by District AYUSH officer while in Maharashtra in Pune district, 13 Ayurvedic dispensaries and 8 Primary Health Units (PHU) are under dual supervision of DHO and Regional Assistant Director AYUSH of Pune region. In Maharashtra co-location is projected in terms of appointment of BAMS doctors in PHCs of remote areas where MBBS are not available. There is no documentation or reports of utilization of Ayurvedic drug kits.

Table 5.15: Spot observations of PHC, in three States: Study districts

State and District	*Chhattisgarh Bilaspur*	*Madhya Pradesh Sagar*	*Himachal Pradesh Hamirpur*
PHC/Block	Kotami (Pendra), Dhobohar (Marwahi)	Tada (Kesali), Dhana (Sagar)	Saloni and Barsar
Doctor	Non-Resident	Resident at Tada	Non-resident at Saloni
Other staff	Adequate, Negative attitude to common people	Adequate: 11.0 am-1.0 pm Negative attitude to common people	Adequate, whole time attendance for OPD
OPD and Records	4-12 pts per day, records not in PHC	4-12 pts per day. Records not in PHC	30-50pts per day. Records in position
AYUSH	No facility	No facility	No facility
Infrastructure	Water scarce/absent OPD room, Store, Delivery room (not maintained) ward, non-functional pathology lab, office. No x-ray machine Operation theatre: no Equipment or facility	Water available OPD room, store, Delivery room (not maintained), ward, non-functioning pathology lab, office x-ray machine absent Operation theatre: no equipment or facility	Water available OPD room, Store, Delivery room (not maintained) ward, pathology lab, Operation theatre: no equipment or facility. X-ray machine absent in Saloni

Source: Research Team's field investigation.

Promotion Policy and Pay Scales of AYUSH Manpower

There are hardly any promotional channels for AYUSH personnel. There also seemed to be wide disparities in the pay scales as compared to Allopathy system. There was a demand for pathology lab instruments and facilities for processing the herbs.

Training and IEC in AYUSH

In training syllabus of ANMs, Anganwadi workers, and ASHA there is absence of AYUSH component. A separate AYUSH nursing college is planned in Himachal Pradesh.

There is a great demand for training in AYUSH from paramedical staff like ANMs, pharmacist and *Dais*. AYUSH doctors are having CMEs in Himachal Pradesh. There is an urgent need for developing training material and publicity material for AYUSH awareness activities in schools, public places, media etc. A well established IEC bureau for AYUSH was felt to be necessary at every State level. It is worth pointing out in this connection that Allopathy doctor's ignorance about AYUSH was colossal and they also needed exposure to CME programmes in AYUSH. Similar situation has been reported from SEDEM and NHSRC studies.

Bed Occupancy in AYUSH Hospitals

Poor bed occupancy in AYUSH hospitals was another striking feature in all the States. There was found to be enough bed space for starting maternity services, which has been lacking at State level or district AYUSH hospitals in all the States. Lack of back up services and facilities like surgical facilities, blood transfusion and anesthesia were the excuses given by the authorities for not starting maternity facility. This problem could be managed by identifying proper referral hospitals and vehicle availability in cases of emergency. Demand for *Panchkarma* and *Kshar-sutra chikitsa* was seen to give distinct visible identity to AYUSH. Several lady AMOs are working in AHCs in all States without any facility for conducting maternity services. Some of them are giving these services at a personal level.

Table 5.16 is an indicator of OPD at co-location at the CHC level and the OPD at the stand-alone AYUSH dispensaries. Rajasthan which has got largest number of AYUSH dispensaries since the time of princely States has the largest turn out at OPD. Large number of AYUSH facilities in Chhattisgarh and Himachal Pradesh is reflected in the large OPD numbers.

Table 5.16: Number of Patients who visited Government Health Care Facilities under AYUSH during 2010-11

Sl. No.	States/Uts	Hospitals (incl. CHCs)		Disp.	PHCs	Total	
		IPD	OPD	OPD	OPD	IPD	OPD 4+5+6
(1)	(2)	(3)	(4)	(5)	(6)	(7)=(3)	(8)
1.	Chhattisgarh	0	183375	4295367	0	0	4478742
2.	Delhi	49330	582180	4070340	0	49330	4652520
3.	Goa	5592	34519	0	0	5592	34519
4.	Himachal Pradesh	49994	462977	4287566	0	49994	4750543
5.	Jammu & Kashmir	713	60410	2436177	0	713	2496587
6.	Kerala	0	13748	155252	0	0	169000
7.	Manipur	248	54044	2665	197518	248	254227
8.	Meghalaya	0	215760	0	131672	0	347432
9.	Mizoram	0	0	51829	0	0	51829
10.	Nagaland	121	10572	575	8161	121	19308
11.	Rajasthan	0	1004077	17220351	0	0	18224428
12.	Tripura	7680	1454432	0	0	7680	1454432
13.	Chandigarh	0	41878	124495	0	0	166373
14.	D & N Haveli	0	0	22931	0	0	22931
15.	Daman & Diu	0	34705	0	5397	0	40102
16.	Puducherry	0	122574	103894	236079	0	462547
	Total	113678	4275251	32771442	578827	113678	37625520

Source: AYUSH in India, 2010: 283.

Primary Health Care Providers

One of the objectives of the study was to study the utilization of AYUSH facilities, OPD attendance, coordination and functional integration with allopathic counterparts, levels of sensitization of various levels of health functionaries regarding the role of AYUSH in public health. Keeping this in view the research team gathered data from CHCs, PHCs, SHCs, AHCs, Anganwadis etc. The findings are as follows:

Classification of Health-Care Providers

(A) Allopathic Health-care Providers

This include CMO at the district level, the district level Government and private hospitals. The Community Health Centres (CHCs) headed by the Block Medical Officers at the tehsil headquarters along with his team of doctors and paramedical workers. The Primary Health Centres (PHCs), headed by a Medical Officer, Health Assistant, ANM, MPW, Dresser, Pharmacists etc. At the village/hamlet level are the ANMs, Anganwadi workers, ASHA/ Mitanins.

(B) AYUSH Health-care Providers

These include the Ayurvedic District Officer, Ayurvedic Medical Officer, *Dai*/Midwife, Compounder etc. at the Ayurvedic dispensaries both in Chhattisgarh and Madhya Pradesh. However in Himachal Pradesh Ayurvedic Health Centres (AHCs) are popular and greater in number than allopathic PHCs. The AHC buildings are better than some of the PHCs. Besides Ayurvedic Physicians, Homoeopaths, Unani doctors also head certain dispensaries in Madhya Pradesh and Chhattisgarh.

Issues Raised by AYUSH Doctors

The research team organized district as well as State level meetings of health care providers. Some of the issues raised by AYUSH doctors with regard to promotion of AYUSH were:

Disease Treatment

They opined that Ayurvedic practitioners can treat following diseases that are not treated by allopaths. These diseases are:

(a) Jaundice
(b) Piles
(c) Malaria
(d) Anaemia
(e) Arthritis
(f) Gynaecological problems
(g) Male infertility
(h) Paralysis
(i) Diabetes
(j) Leucorrhoea etc.

They firmly said that Ayurveda has medicines/provisions for pre-natal, antenatal and post-natal care as well.

One of the Ayurvedic doctors presented his views by emphasizing on the issues given below:

(a) ***Promoting health education*** among the common masses of village India for positive health.
(b) ***Production and marketing of medicinal herbs***: He emphasized that, production and marketing is one of the most significant aspects of development of Ayurveda. Cultivation of medicinal herbs, their preservation in the forest zones is the need of the hour. He also mentioned Madhya Pradesh has 71,526 villages out of which 30,000 villages are forest villages. The tribal and rural folk of these villages should be associated with cultivation and production of Ayurvedic medicine as an income generation venture.
(c) ***Research and Development***: Today's Ayurveda cannot be compared with the Ayurveda of Charak, Sushrut's time. There is a need to address the demand and current needs, promote research and development in Ayurveda.
   - *Supply of Medicine*: Doctors said they did not get the medicines which they demanded for. The quality of drugs sometimes is not up to the mark.
   - *AYUSH Facilities*: There was a common suggestion that AYUSH facilities should be promoted in all the PHCs.
   - *Infrastructure Facilities in Ayurvedic dispensaries*: During the district and State level meetings the Ayurvedic Physicians expressed following views about infrastructure facilities in Ayurvedic Dispensaries of Madhya Pradesh and Chhattisgarh:
     (a) *Vehicle*: The District Ayurvedic Officer does not have a vehicle to visit and monitor the Ayurvedic Dispensaries. This has created a big gap between the Medical Officers and the DAO.
     (b) *Furniture*: Lack of furniture in the dispensaries was yet another issue.
     (c) *Equipments*: Lack of medical equipments in the dispensaries is a genuine problem that hinders the growth of AYUSH.

(d) *Storage*: Lack of fridge and cupboards for storing medicines is a major hurdle in the dispensaries.

NHSRC report has discussed the "Perceptions of the Health Service Providers Regarding AYUSH and LHT".

Allopathic Doctors

The Allopathic Doctors were generally quite supportive of AYUSH systems. 70 per cent (66 of 94) perceived them as useful, while the rest thought they were redundant and unscientific. Over half of the Allopaths, 55 per cent, perceived value in home remedies and suggested that such practices must be documented, scientifically studied and revived.

Auxiliary Nurse Midwives

All the ANMs interviewed across the States were unaware of public AYUSH services for referring cases, except Tamil Nadu where 25 per cent of the VHNs were trained in ISM, had medicines in their kit and were also referring cases to public AYUSH facilities. However, 52 per cent of the ANMs admitted use of home remedies in minor ailments for themselves and families.

Accredited Social Health Activists

The ASHAs had little awareness of the AYUSH public facilities in the area, except for Odisha and Kerala where the awareness was 60 per cent and 100 per cent, respectively. This was despite them knowing the 1-2 AYUSH remedies they had in their kit, e.g. Ayurvedic drug for anaemia. *Punarnavadi Mandoor* was among a few mentioned in their kit in Odisha and Tamil Nadu.

However, 60 per cent of them did know of local home remedies. Some of them used these remedies in their own families, but did not prescribe them to patients, as in Uttarakhand. Others prescribed them to patients in the community, as in Bihar, Odisha and Tamil Nadu. Hence, in general, ASHAs were unaware of AYUSH services but, to some extent, were using home remedies for their families and sometimes for patients.

Almost all ASHAs (90-100%) were aware of medicinal plants in 12 States, 70 per cent in 2 States, 50-65 per cent in 3 States, and 10 per cent in Kerala; though they were of the opinion that proper use of the medicinal plants is not known to them. ASHAs suggested that generating more awareness on AYUSH and LHT would be useful for the community (NHSRC, 2010: 120-122).

SEDEM (Rajasthan Report) has also discussed the perceptions of AYUSH head of the facilities.

Sample size: 181 AYUSH heads were interviewed: 6 from medical colleges, 24 from district hospitals, 27 from CHCs, 50 from PHCs and 74 from AYUSH dispensaries. All the facilities are co-located except the dispensaries. Not all facilities had a qualified medical physician; these centres were somehow functioning.

Types of Diseases/Conditions Treated at the Institution

Common diseases treated at these institutions are: Diarrhoea, fever, skin diseases, and anaemia (among children), Fever, diarrhoea, joint pain, skin diseases, piles etc. (among adult males), Gynaecological problems, diarrhoea, fever, anaemia, etc. (among adult females) and joint pain, fever, asthma, diarrhoea etc. (among the elderly).

Commonly used Systems

Children: Exclusively AYUSH is used for treating fever (84%), Diarrhoea (75%), skin diseases (14%), and anaemia (13%).

Adult Males: Exclusively AYUSH is used by 72 per cent for treating fever, 62 per cent for treating diarrhoea, 27 per cent for treating joint pain, and 19 per cent each for treating asthma and skin diseases.

Adult Females: Exclusively AYUSH is used by 76 per cent for treating gynaecological disorders, 49 per cent for treating fever, 37 per cent for treating diarrhoea, 15 per cent for treating joint pain, 10 per cent for treating skin diseases.

The Elderly: Exclusively AYUSH is used by 51 per cent for treating Asthma, by 57 per cent for treating joint pain, by 48 per cent for treating fever, by 44 per cent for treating diarrhoea, 12 per cent for anaemia, 11 per cent for ENT disorders, and by 8 per cent for treating skin disorders.

Referral Systems (Cross-system)

According to 66.3 per cent of the sample AYUSH doctors, cases from allopathic system are referred to AYUSH doctors. 33.7 per cent say that this sort of referral does not occur.

According to the doctors the top five diseases in which allopaths referred cases to AYUSH system included: Diarrhoea, joint pain, skin diseases, piles and certain gynaecological problems. Doctors who resort to cross-referral include cases of diarrhoea (18%), skin diseases and joint pain (14% for each), piles (11%), and gynaecological problems (9%). These five diseases account for 65 per cent of total referrals as stated by AYUSH head of the facilities.

Seventy nine per cent of the doctors interviewed say that cases coming to AYUSH are referred to allopathic system, should it be required. 21 per cent say that cases are not referred.

Instances of cross-referrals occur in cases of injury (29%), fever (17%), TB (14%), diarrhoea (11%) and gynaecological problems (7%). Of the total responses, 77 per cent of cross-referred cases are accounted for by these five ailments.

ASHA and AYUSH Component within NRHM

Nearly 85 per cent AYUSH doctors say that no AYUSH specific components have been included for ASHA. Responses from ASHA interviewed at Ajmer indicate that they don't promote LHT or home remedies; they simply carry the kits and dispense what they should. The user groups also confirm that ASHA do not normally recommend home remedies or promote LHT. Very few doctors responded in the affirmative that AYUSH components have been included in ASHA's training module (SEDEM 2010: 25-31).

It is quite clear that AYUSH in public sector does not really exists functionally in comparison to the PHC system which is dominated in all forms by allopathy. AHCs in reality are the dispensaries providing curative medicine in a referral mode to home remedies or medicine given by herbalist. Paradoxically, the health workers who are closest to people, by their upbringing and by their professional requirements, are linked formally to PHC upward hierarchical system and not to AYUSH, which is their rightful place. NRHM's idealism of co-location cannot be made operational by administrative or legislative regulations, unless matched by overall medical education in favour of AYUSH, at the medical schools and more importantly at the para-medical schools which are far less in number. India does not require more doctors for primary health care but more para-professionals and an army of volunteers of women who are oriented to plural systems of health care, including the fair amount of stadardisation of home remedies. We also need to incorporate the traditional herbalists and *dai* with continuous upscaling of their skills and knowledge of AYUSH systems and acumen to refer the cases upwards when necessary.

Public Perception

When people introduce the village to a guest, they say, "this is our temple, our school, our meeting place, *chaupal-chavdi* and that (PHC) is the Government health centre". When I asked villagers as to who constructed a beautiful temple in the heart of the village, proudly they said, "We did it, with our funds. We went to Jaipur to select a marble icon of the deity. We keep the temple clean." To a question as to why there was an open drain outside the temple over which one had to jump to enter the temple, they said, it was for the Government to do it.

6
PRIVATE SECTOR
Health Care Market

Before the Government established PHC, SC and AHC, all health care was in the domain of families, kin group, neighbourhood and village community. In the pre-industrial urban centres, there were professionally trained Vaidya and Hakims trained by the Gurus or within the family. They were available only as referral physicians. All citizens were looked after in the folk tradition of home remedies blessed by local healers who had indigenous knowledge of herbal, mineral or animal-fish medicine and by the *Dais* specialising on reproductive and child health. The folk traditions continue mostly in rural and tribal areas. These are not conventionally called as private sector since the local healers or *Dais* do not fix standard payment for services rendered. They are paid in cash and kind by the people voluntarily depending upon the paying capacity of the beneficiary family. Professional services have been rendered by these healers by way of helping fellow citizens in a group of villages or kin or neighbours, not for consideration as the case with professional clinicians or chemists.

Private Sector in health as it functions on the ground particularly in the rural areas refer to all those persons, trained or untrained, who offer their knowledge or skills for diagnosing a malady when approached and offer treatment for which regular fee is charged. Many doctors, ANMs, chemists, other paramedics as compounders, who while employed in the public sector also run private clinics during or after office hours. There are others who are wholly doing private practice. Some of them are doctors with graduation in any system of medicine. Others irrespective of their formal qualification, who may be referred to as quacks in the formal health care terminology, are addressed as doctors by the patients who seek their services.

Once while undertaking fieldwork with Prof. Peltoan, American Medical Anthropologist in a village in Vallabhgarh (Ballabhgarh) internship training area under All India Institute of Medical Sciences, New Delhi, on behalf of the Ford Foundation, we interviewed a clinician who became doctor on the strength of his experience as a compounder for 15 years with a senior doctor. He had gone to treat a case of acute diarrhoea keeping us waiting for some time. On return, he said diarrhoea was caused by insects at the root of cauliflower and he treated the cases successfully. How does it matter about his cause-effect knowledge as long as he could provide relief to the patient? Even in a city, like Pune, we have seen a mechanic from ammunition factory who would treat his patients with an injection, or even a qualified doctor who had nothing in his urban clinic except the equipment for boiling injection needles, no pieces of furniture except a table to keep a stove. He spent one hour in that clinic every evening.

At Rajnandgon village in Chhattisgarh, a PMW in leprosy who visited a leprosy patient to monitor his MDT, in his official capacity, reported his private practice which earned for him atleast Rs. 100 per day besides his government salary. On the particular day of our presence, he gave a B-complex injection to a woman complaining weakness and reportedly charged Rs. 10.

On the other hand, a Professor of Obstetrics and Gynaecology at a government medical college was summoned to the palace of the princely State to assist the delivery of the Queen, who gave birth to the Prince. On inquiry, she said, she received heavy gold necklace and an expensive saree as a gift, not as payment. I asked her as to how was she different from a *Dai* performing in a village family getting a *saree* and some grain by way of voluntary consideration.

Field investigations in Madhya Pradesh, Chhattisgarh, Himachal Pradesh and Maharashtra have provided data about private sector in Health.

Chhattisgarh: About 14 private practitioners were interviewed in Perndra (8) and Marwahi (6) blocks.

Homoeopathic Doctors felt people had inclination for allopathy. They had no awareness about Homoeopathy. Ayurvedic practitioners felt about the side effects of allopathic drugs. They recommended integration of all systems at the PHC, District and State level hospitals. One private practitioner, age 27 practices in at least four villages. He keeps medicines for fever, diarrhoea, dysentery, malaria, general debility etc. He also administers IV glucose. He treats about 8-10 patients every day and earns Rs. 50-100 per patient.

A tribal quack doctor, age 39 years educated 12 standard, was working as a community health worker for 7 years. He works in a radius of about 5-6 km villages. In a month, he treated 25 patients of cough-cold, 30 for fever, 10 for boils and other skin conditions and 10 patients complaining stomach problems. A chemist owning a pharmacy shop generally practices allopathy but keeps ayurvedic and unani drugs in the shop like Jalimloshan, Noorani oil etc. He claims, more patients with viral fever seek his help. Another grocery shop owner keeps some common allopathic drugs like Paracetamol, Metranidazole, Albendagole, Lomofin, ORS, Diclovin, Aciloc etc. None of the two shop keepers know anything about AYUSH.

In Himachal Pradesh, the doctors working in the public sector practice at home in the evening. But they remain at the AHC as per government rules. None of them are resident doctors at the AHC as there are no residential quarters for the doctors in Hamirpur district. In Himachal the villages are developed in comparison to those in Madhya Pradesh or Chhattisgarh. So, the doctors' houses in the villages are quite spacious to allow them to do private practice. Many doctors live in nearby towns and daily commute to their respective AHC in their cars.

It appears there are more quacks and paramedics doing private practice in the villages in the States.

Private Doctors and Health Practitioners

The private doctors visit the village once or twice in a week and some of them have regular patients in these villages who take treatment for chronic illnesses.

There are BAMS doctors too who run their private clinics and prescribe both Allopathic and Ayurvedic medicines to the villagers. Several such clinics and pharmacy shops are visible at the tehsil headquarters, which are visited by the peasantry from neighbouring villages, while they visit the towns for marketing. Several quakes are also seen practicing at the weekly markets.

These private practitioners prescribe medicines to pregnant women on the basis of their symptoms and do not carry out a physical examination on them. Most of the times the pregnant women in the villages consult the ANM or the lady doctor at the PHC and if the PHC is not present in the villages, they consult the AWW or ASHA who help them with their immunisation and provide them with iron tablets. It is only in rare cases that the pregnant women consult private doctors in the villages.

Other than the private doctors, the villagers believe in self-medication and most of the households purchase over-the-counter medicines such as Saridon, Nimucilide, Paracetamol, tonics etc. People generally do not go to the district hospital but prefer to consult the BAMS or allopathic doctors at private hospitals who provide medicines from both the systems of medicine irrespective of the system they have been trained in. As a result the private doctors are in demand and have a good practice in the villages.

Some unqualified graduate degree holders have opened dispensaries in nearby villages and treat patients with Allopathy or Ayurvedic medicines which include eye drops, tonics and medicines for diarrhoea, vomiting, fever etc. For emergencies they go for home visits. They also provide medicines such as Liv-52, Safi, and various tonics etc. to the villagers. These private clinics have examination tables and intra-venous drip facilities.

Chemists

There were 6 medical stores in the Madhya Pradesh study area. Interviews with owners revealed that the chemist shops store both Allopathic and Ayurvedic medicines like Drakshasav, Kankasav, Ashwagandharishta, Dashmularishta, Dabur laaltel, Chyawanprasha, Pudinhara, Amritarishta, Baal Jeevanghutti, Gripewater, Spaki, Liv-52, Tentex Royal, Mental Agro Red Oil, Kumariasav, Systone tablet, Martand Salt, Ashokarishta, Hingwahtak Churna, Lavanbhaskarchurna, Mahanarayan Oil, Hempushpa, Shankhapushpi, Pathyadikadha, M-2 Tone etc.

The medicines prescribed by the private BAMS doctors are all available in these pharmacies. All the medicines and injections prescribed by the Medical Officer at the PHC are generally not available at the PHC but can be bought at these pharmacies.

The villagers take over-the-counter medicines from the chemist after telling him the symptoms. The chemist suggests the medicines accordingly. Most common among these are Lomofen (commonly known as yellow tablet) and Entrequinol (commonly known as green tablet) which are bought by the village elders as well as the children directly from the chemist shop. Villagers also buy Ayurvedic preparations from companies such as Baidyanath and Dabur as the packaging of these preparations and drugs contain directions for use, indications and symptoms written in Hindi and regional language, which facilitates its use.

- Dhana PHC MO prescribes tonics and injections not available in PHC for purchase from medical stores located at 1 km distance.
- Private BAMS doctors prescribe nearly 25 types of ayurvedic medicines which are available in local shops.
- Ayurved dispensary MO also writes prescriptions
- Doctor from Sanaudhaayurvedic dispensary has good reputation for giving cure to 100 per cent patients with Ayurved as well as Allopathy medicines.

Recommendations by Chemists

- Village people do not have enough awareness and knowledge about Ayurved, but can be promoted through training.
- Doctors themselves do not use ayurvedic drugs.
- Ayurved drugs are costly.
- Not available in small packs.
- Doctors should prescribe Ayurved.
- Quality of drugs should improve.
- There should be a resident doctor in the village.

As per other medical stores owner, he sells 80 per cent Ayurved and 20 per cent Allopathy drugs as one RMP doctor treats patients with Ayurved drugs and also prescribes Ayurved medicines. RMP doctors use both systems, but promote Ayurved, thinking they were safe and acceptable to people by taste and flavour.

Drug production companies have commercial interests and prepare substandard drugs. There are low quality components in some combinations, e.g. Shitopaladi Churna contains impure Vanshlochan which is not effective. Similarly, tablet Niri's composition is wrong according to texts.

(A) Chemists and Pharmacists

It was observed in all the four States that chemists and pharmacists especially in the villages gave medicines for common ailments. In many places some of them are believed to function like doctors.

(B) Grocery Shops and Pan Stall Owners

In Madhya Pradesh we observed grocery shop and Pan Stall owners selling *"Mathura Pudis"*, i.e. powdered Aspirin for one rupee for headache/cold. These are very popular for quick relief.

(C) Quack

In all the four States we observed quacks who practice as doctors, in the weekly markets, in their own clinics, at home or they visit villages daily to call on the patients.

(D) Private Doctors

BAMS, BHMS, MBBS doctors were also seen practicing in the villages under study, usually referred to as motorcycle doctors as they visited the villages on specific days of the week for few hours.

Ayurvedic Drug Stores: The villages having A.H.C.s had one or two Ayurvedic drug stores. In Gahaliya (Himachal Pradesh), a chemist was interviewed. He said the villagers preferred Ayurvedic medicines and hence over 70 per cent of the medicines in his store are Ayurvedic. In the absence of A.H.C. doctor, the villagers avail Ayurvedic medicines from the drug store. The store owner has a good rapport with A.H.C. doctor and is aware of most medicines prescribed by the A.H.C. doctor for certain common ailments.

Chemist Shops

There are 8 medical stores opposite CHC Barsar, Hamirpur district.

- All 3 chemists had a degree in pharmacy.

- On an average all the 3 chemists had 200 different types of medicines.
- About 60-75 per cent of their total number of medicines were allopathic as per allopathic CHC.
- About 10-20 per cent of the purchasers preferred to buy Ayurvedic medicines.
- All the three medical stores get their medicines from Hamirpur and Una.
- All the three chemists said that production of allopathic as well as Ayurvedic medicines takes place in factories of Solan and more precisely in a place called Baddi, which is an industrial hub.
- In the vicinity of AHC, the drug stores sell about 80 per cent Ayurvedic drugs and 20 per cent Allopathic drugs.

Doctors' Observations about AYUSH

1. Ayurved treatment is definitely better and effective and it has no side effects.
2. Ayurved medicines should be available in small packs and packed like Allopathy medicines and in small sizes.
3. Some AYUSH doctors give symptomatic treatment and do not treat the rootcause.
4. Government Ayurvedic Doctors use injections and allopathy drugs even if they have Ayurvedic drugs available for treatment.
5. Ayurved doctor of Ayurved dispensary Bamghari said that there is no proper place and facilities for treating patients. His clinic is currently run in Panchayat Bhavan. People from nearby villages come for treatment.
6. In Laghori AHC only couple of patients come per day. The doctor keeps the medicine stock at home. AHC is managed by pharmacist as patients don't go there. In his opinion patient wants quick relief while Ayurved drugs take time and are slow.
7. According to them some Ayurvedic medicines such as *Musli* powder available in the market are expensive and not of such a good quality. It's better to process them at home as they will be of a better quality and inexpensive too.

8. The Ayurvedic injections such as *'Bel'* or garlic injections are ineffective.
9. Ayurveda doesn't have any side effects, hence it should be promoted.
10. The packaging of the Ayurvedic medicines should be done similarly to allopathic medicines and the packaging should be smaller in size.
11. Ayurvedic doctors should conduct proper diagnosis of the patients before giving them medicines.
12. Ayurvedic doctors prescribe both allopathic and Ayurvedic medicines. They have adequate Ayurvedic drugs which they should prescribe and use.
13. There is a need for good buildings with proper facilities, adequate medicines and availability of staff quarters.

Private sector functioning in the villages all over the country provides a common scenario. Proliferation of medical colleges of all systems of dubious standards do not provide services of professionally trained doctors to the villagers. The LCPS and LMP short courses were more popular in pre-independence days as there were very few medical colleges in the country.

In the recent past, attempts to start shorter diploma courses in medicine to suit the requirements of rural sector met with opposition from the medical personnel of all systems of medicine. Good qualitative or quantitative studies are not available about the private sector. Smart para-medics have good private practice in rural India.

7
STAKEHOLDER PRESCRIPTIONS

People have stakes in health. They want to remain healthy to be able to perform social roles as per their ascribed and achieved statuses within the homes and in the community. Cultural practices are tuned to preserve and promote health by way of nutrition, diet, rest and work as per occupation. The gender and age differences are organized in social structure.

Any event of disequilibrium with the environment or daily schedule of living at the physical or mental level could lead to discomfort which might need corrective action. Culturally and socially accepted traditional home remedies using the herbs normally used as kitchen condiments provide relief or prevents further discomfiture. If not manageable, local traditional herbalists or more knowledgeable elders are available for consultation. In some cases, spiritual or ritualistic remedies are sought as alternative or complementary therapies.

The concept of welfare state has enjoined upon the Government to provide facilities in the public sector about health care. Immunization for prevention of epidemics of communicable diseases are available. Institutionalization of health care in rural India with holistic concepts of rural or community development initiated in 1952 required professionally trained medical and paramedical personnel to deliver health care facilities. During historical times, more particularly in the princely States, during British Rule, traditional Indian systems such as Ayurved, Unani and Siddha were promoted in the capital towns for training of medical personnel and dispensing of drugs.

As a social sector activity, in a democratic electoral process, health care and expanding opportunities for formal education are the two visible welfare activities promoted by all political parties.

As a result the facilities and medical-paramedical manpower has been steadily increasing. All these personnel are also stakeholders in health care delivery. The plural systems of medicine historically evolved in India have given rise to parallel institutional structures with ensured autonomy. So, there are medical personnel functioning in the respective medical systems. For some of the national level health care programmes such as MCH, RCH family planning, disease control programmes as in Malaria, Leprosy etc. medical and paramedical personnel have been appointed. A balance has to be struck between professionally trained doctors and paramedics who actually deliver the services at the doorstep of the people. All these quantitative expansions in a short period after Independence pose issues of networking, co-ordination and convergence at various levels of political decision making and hierarchical administrative services with powers, obligations and funds divided between the Central and State governments in a federal system. These are all stakeholders in health care.

To streamline the issues and more towards co-ordination among the plural systems, with a genuine desire to provide the strengths of each system to the citizens, National Rural Health Mission was established. It, however, appears that the lofty ideal of co-location has been functioning in different styles in different States of India.

The qualitative studies by MAAS in four States of India, viz., Himachal Pradesh, Madhya Pradesh, Chhattisgarh and Maharashtra required establishing close rapport with the people in selected villages, among the paramedics and medics. This was possible by following the anthropological method of participant observation, informal key interviews, focused group discussions etc. by living with the people in the families and villages under study. As an ethical practice, it is also necessary to discuss the observations with the study participant people. This resulted in the organization of mixed group meetings. The observations were also shared with the administrators and politicians through these meetings, the details of which have been documented. On earlier occasions, informal discussions were held with the groups of persons holding a similar position, such as the Anganwadi, ANM, doctors etc. At each such meeting the participants made operational suggestions to improve the quality of services and to ensure co-ordination amongst all health workers in the interests of people's health.

Stakeholder's consultative meetings of staff of AYUSH Health Centres, e.g. AYUSH medical officers and paramedical staff, e.g. midwives and pharmacist, AYUSH block level and district level officers, medical officers of PHC/CHC, ANMs, Anganwadi workers, ASHA, local health care functionaries like *Dais* and herbalist from the study area were held at the district or block place followed by state level meetings with State authorities in each state. The idea of these meetings was to discuss the issues about Mainstreaming of AYUSH in Public Health in a free atmosphere keeping aside one's work-place designations and hierarchies. All these meetings were initiated as a part of study methodology.

The meetings were held in each state but the best meetings were in Himachal Pradesh where along with health functionaries the elected representatives from block level were also present in block level meeting and for the first time health functionaries of various categories from Government sector of Ayurved and Allopathy and people's sector were called together at block level to discuss openly the issue of mainstreaming of AYUSH in public health. The participants discussed about their concerns and gaps at organization and infrastructure levels which need to be attended for promoting AYUSH. Each participant specifically said that such joint meetings were very necessary for frequent interactions to improve health services. They said, they had met first time like this without a formal agenda and could speak freely without any reservations.

Minister of Health and Ayurved of Himachal Pradesh who was an Ayurved physician presided over the state level meeting. He made 3 important points:

- He asked the study team to advise on mainstreaming home practices in health care.
- He advised the AYUSH doctors from AYUSH Health Centres that preventive health care and IEC work in their area was their job responsibility and not only attending OPD.
- He also advised not to compare AYUSH with Allopathic system.

Table 7.1: Details of Stakeholders Consultative Meetings convented by project investigation

Sl. No.	*State*	*Date*	*Time Duration of meeting and Participants*	*Place*
1. Himachal Pradesh				
(i)	District Level	27/6/09	Allopathic and AYUSH Doctors, ANM, AWW, Pharmacist, Midwife, Z.P. Member, P.S.-Chairman Participants 40 Duration 3½ hrs	Mehere–Barsar, Government Guest House
(ii)	State Level	30/6/09	Hon. Minister of Health and Ayurved, Secretary, Director of Ayurved—OSD (Projects) Shimla, Representative of Director of Health NRHM, AYUSH doctors Participants 15 Duration 1 Hr.	Secretariat Shimla
2. Madhya Pradesh				
(i)	District Level	19/5/09	District Ayurved Officer, AYUSH Doctors Duration 2 Hrs..Participants 19	Sagar University
(ii)	State Level	15/6/09	Commissioner, Dy. Directors District Officer Duration 1 Hr. Participants 4	Bhopal Commissioner's Chamber
3. Chhattisgarh				
(i)	District + State Level meeting	23/5/09	Director of Ayurved, OSD Retired Director of Health DAO, Bilaspur, AYUSH Doctors from the field SHSRC AYUSH Doctor Duration 2 Hrs. Participants 11	Raipur Directorate of AYUSH
4. Maharashtra				
(i)	District Level	6/6/09	1. SHSRC Director for 2 hrs. Participants 6	Pune
(ii)	State Level	28/7/09	2. Jt. Secy. Public Health, Dir. SHSRC, Asst. Dir. (AYU), NGO, AYU Medical College and Tribal Herbalist, Dr. Arole Duration 2½ Hrs. Participants 20	SHSRC

Source: Research Team's field investigation.

- The other participants at Shimla meeting were the Secretary of Health, NRHM Director, Director and OSD for AYUSH, Himachal Pradesh, co-ordinator of MAAS project etc.

The district meeting at Sagar, Madhya Pradesh discussed about motivation of AYUSH doctors. Chhattisgarh meeting was attended by retired Director of Health Services. At Pune, retired Director of Health Services who is the current Director of SHSRC and Joint Secretary, Health Services were present.

The following paragraphs give the AYUSH health care requirements as suggested by the participants at various levels. Important points that emerged from these meetings and the recommendations:

- IEC and general awareness activities about AYUSH to be planned for people at community level to inform about the strengths of all AYUSH systems so that people can exercise their choice of treatment system.
- For co-location strategy of facilities, there was general agreement. The Allopathic doctors from PHC and CHC were particularly in favour of co-location as it would facilitate availability of more doctors and sharing of responsibility for emergencies and medico-legal cases from AYUSH doctors.
- Plural therapy and cross therapy to be consciously promoted at AYUSH co-location.
- Cross referral and co-ordination be made mandatory in some form to avoid duplication. In each of the district Ayurved hospitals in Himachal Pradesh, homoeopathy clinics are located. But it was observed that both Ayurved as well as homoeopathy doctors claimed a cure for all problems in their system and did not practice cross referral. Ayurved doctors were seen to practice Allopathy instead of referring and allopathy doctors were also using branded Ayurved drugs.
- Doctor's demand for training: AYUSH doctors suggested to have training in emergency care through Continuing Medical Education (CME) while Allopathy doctors desired CME for facilitating cross referrals.

- The knowledge of all AYUSH systems and their respective strengths should be known to all AYUSH as well as Allopathy doctors and paramedical staff.
- Health statistics of AYUSH work and their health care share in the state is not included in the yearly official state level health publication (Health at a Glance). One civil services AYUSH Director said that they are subordinate junior partners and do not get credit for their work in national programmes. AYUSH contribution in implementation of national programmes was not acknowledged in the state report in Himachal Pradesh. The credit is taken away by health department.
- Coordination of plural systems at block and district level has to be formalized by way of quarterly meetings.
- In AYUSH dispensaries AYUSH doctors are said to be underutilized by AYUSH as they manage only OPD. They are utilized for school health checkups during certain months and for mass polio immunization programmes. School Health Survey and AYUSH IEC could be linked.
- Special national programmes based on AYUSH strengths could be started with AYUSH as a nodal agency, e.g. Anaemia Free Himachal, geriatric care, *Ksharsutra Chikitsa, Panchkarma,* and maternal and child health.
- AYUSH Health camps, e.g. *Ksharsutra* in Himachal Pradesh were seen to help image building and develop distinct identity to AYUSH.
- In Chhattisgarh, schemes like Ayurved gram and God Grahita gram are initiatives of AYUSH Department.
- There was a demand for AYUSH sub-centres on lines of PHC, specially in Himachal Pradesh.
- AHCs to have attached residential quarters for AYUSH doctors.
- Physicians and paramedical workers to be encouraged for AYUSH tourism.
- AYUSH day to be celebrated by Ministry of Health.
- AYUSH doctor/AHC doctor be asked to supervise the work of SC and anganwadi in AHC village and in the nighbourhood.

Demands and Suggestions from Paramedical Personnel

- Demand for co-location of AHC at PHC sub-centre and Anganwadi level was more from ANMs for reasons of coordinated activities and to have sub-centres open when ANM are on field visits. Coincidental co-location of AHC, Sub-centre and Anganwadi at Gahaliya village in Himachal Pradesh is very effective in providing services.
- Anaemia control programme in Himachal under AYUSH is going on with coordination of all health functionaries.
- ANMs desired training in AYUSH, so that, they can communicate with local herbalist.
- Mitanin in Chhattisgarh is equivalent to ASHA. Mitanins are bound to families as friends in need at hamlet level which is the unit of social action and need to be initiated in health system for better results. Mitanins are trained in home remedies which brings Mitanins in closer contact with herbalists/Baiga. Monthly meetings with villagers are reported by Mitanins in study villages for local networking.
- PHC Sub-centre and Anganwadi could become the hub of women activities and respective places used for the whole day if such meetings are coordinated by AYUSH Doctor or Sarpanch or Secretary.
- ASHA requires AYUSH IEC material for Mahila Mandals.
- *AYUSH drug kits:* AYUSH drugs were not seen in ASHA/ Mitanin kits. ASHA and Mitanin kits should contain AYUSH drugs and kit supply should be regular.

Training Needs

- Frequent training to ASHA/Mitanin in AYUSH can be arranged by SHSRC through NRHM. Training of ASHA in AYUSH though mentioned in syllabus is missing in practice and needs strengthening.
- AWWs demanded proper training to use medicine kits given to them through ICDS. AWW used to get AYUSH medicine kits from ICDS without getting training for using these medicines. In their personal lives, AWW prefer home remedies before trying medicines from their kits.

- Anganwadi worker desired AYUSH training to help women and children and also for communicating with local herbalists.
- AWW desired for training in nutrition, diets, home remedies and AYUSH based Mother and Child care. AYUSH based diets and supplementation could be designed based on local conditions and availability.
- All untrained *Dais* demanded training which could be imparted by AYUSH doctors.
- Herbalist's training for 2 weeks to be designed by Department of AYUSH and participation certificate to be given.
- Demands and suggestions from Government pharmacists were important and were as follows:
    (a) To streamline the gaps in central drug supplies as there is mismatch between requirement of specific drugs and what is supplied.
    (b) To provide instruments/utensils in AHCs for processing of drugs from herbs in coordination with local herbalist, e.g. making fresh decoctions of herbs. Pharmacist showed willingness to train herbalists to make drugs.
    (c) Pharmacists and doctors recommend supply of Ayurvedic drugs in small and attractive packing to avoid dispensing in small loose shabby paper wrapping.
- Village representatives in Himachal Pradesh expressed concern about quality of some AYUSH drugs.
- Plantations of medicinal plants was recommended by village people in Himachal Pradesh and in Chhattisgarh in Ayurved gram.
- Chemist shops keep both allopathy and Ayurvedic drugs. The sale varies from 20 to 70 per cent. Ayurved doctors prescribe Allopathy drugs for faster relief. Women after delivery use Ayurvedic medicines.

Health Infrastructure Recommendations from Stakeholders Meeting

- All district level AYUSH hospitals should have a maternity ward.

- AHC should have ANC/PNC facilities.
- Minimum facilities such as Water, Electricity, Telephone and equipments should be there in PHCs, Sub-centres and Ayurved dispensaries.
- Physical presence of medical and paramedical staff in PHCs, SCs and Ayurved dispensaries is essential.
- OPD timings should be from 8 am to 1 pm instead of 11 am to 1 pm.
- AYUSH room with doctors and medicines should be available in all PHCs, SCs and Ayurved dispensaries.
- Ayurvedic dispensaries to be given PHC status and should have SCs to popularize and promote AYUSH at grassroots level.
- Healthy coordination between PHC, ICDS and AYUSH staff at all levels is essential.
- Co-location of AYUSH and PHC is essential.
- Baiga (herbalists), masseurs and bone setters should be part of health care system.
- Both CHCs and AYUSH health care providers should jointly get involved in preparing training material on AYUSH for Mitanin, Baiga/Vaidu, Aaganwadi workers and TBAs.
- Ayurved Gram and Godgrahita Gram: IEC work to AYUSH Doctors and monitoring of Medicinal Plantation on village common lands.
- What about monitoring by District AYUSH authorities without transport?
- Mitanin Training—Home Remedies. Contact with Herbalist—Baiga.
- Demand for AYUSH training and AYUSH drugs by ANM, ASHA, Mitanin, AWW.
- Ayurved Gram in Chhattisgarh, to be activated for plantation on individual and village lands: role of PRI.
- Demand for AYUSH IEC material.
- AWW demand AYUSH training in nutritious diet and household medicine, and AYUSH drugs.
- Home remedies could be standardized at the level of AHC in consultation with Village Health and Sanitation Committee.

- Fair price or minimum price has to guaranteed for medicinal herbs.
- Kitchen branded condiments are advertised widely. They could promote medicinal qualities of these herbs.
- Primary Health Care publications from AYUSH perspectives are needed.
- Tamil Nadu Government had advertised in newspapers about medicinal herbs for preventing, protecting against Dengue and Swine Flu. This needs to be followed by other State Governments.
- Iron tablets given to pregnant women under ANC care are widely rejected. Equivalent AYUSH products along with nutritional advice for iron intake can be given. These could be grown in kitchen gardens or in balconies, open spaces in the compound.
- Untied funds to DAO, MO, and AHC for quick action.
- Social audit by village health and sanitation committee.

Dai/TBA Recommendations from Chhattisgarh

- They want to work in hospitals.
- Trained *dais* want refresher training.
- They want themselves to be attached officially with ANMs so that they can help in deliveries.
- Untrained *Dais* need to be trained by PHCs and AYUSH personnel.
- Delivery kit to be supplied regularly and monitored.
- Many *Dais* expressed their desire for incentives in cash or kind.
- *Dais* were interested in getting training from Government sector and suggested to include information about medicinal plants or herbs which can be used by them after delivery.

Baiga Recommendations from Chhattisgarh

- They do not want their knowledge to fade away for want of official recognition and support.
- To expand their traditional knowledge, they want frequent trainings from Ayurved doctors.

- Training for identification and processing of medicinal plants to prepare medicines is needed and it should be near their village.
- Training of Baigas on AYUSH lines and incorporating their services in primary health care given through Ayurved dispensaries is the need of Chhattisgarh herbal state.
- Every panchayat should have a land reserved for growing medicinal plants and Baigas of the village should be trained and given the responsibility to maintain and monitor the growth of these plants.
- Monthly village level meetings to disseminate the traditional knowledge of Baigas to the people.
- Baigas should have AYUSH medicines.
- Educated Youths of the village should be trained in AYUSH and encouraged to cultivate medicinal plants on mass scale.
- Specialist Baigas should receive more attention for training and improvement of their skills. Their services during birthing process are important.
- Directory and documentation of their knowledge is essential.

Baiga's Opinions

- According to them, Ayurved needs to be promoted by creating awareness among the people. Unless the people are aware about it, it would not get the standing it deserves.
- Locals who can recognize the herbs or have knowledge about the herbs can be useful in creating awareness in the community for promotion of Ayurved.
- Need for update about knowledge about herbs and processing was expressed.

Recommendations by Anganwadis

- The AWWs should be provided with equipments such as blood pressure machine, stethoscope etc. and they should be properly trained in using these equipments.
- They should be trained about the use and benefits of Ayurvedic medicines and they should in turn train the

members of the various women's groups in the same.

- The workers at the Anganwadis wanted to be trained in AYUSH related health practices and such training should be provided to them.
- AYUSH related nutritional supplements should be included in the nutritious food supplied at the Anganwadis.

Recommendations of PHC Allopathic Medical Officers

- PHCs running in sub-centre buildings need urgent attention.
- Vacant posts need to be filled.
- Beds, generators, X-ray machines, vehicles need to be made available.
- Co-location for AYUSH treatments should have separate room.

Recommendations of Ayurved Doctors of Ayurved Health Centres

- Ayurved dispensaries should have Government buildings.
- Doctors want residential quarters near Ayurved dispensary.
- Staff vacancies to be filled.
- Frequent CME programmes to get update on Ayurved research and advances.
- Ayurved drug supply to be provided in small packs for easy dispensing.
- Ayurved to be popularized in villages with the help of posters and slogans.

ANM Recommendations

- Sub-centre building and residential quarters should be there.
- They should receive training about AYUSH and Ayurvedic drugs.
- At sub-centre, Allopathic and Ayurvedic drugs should be available.

- Sub-centre to be equipped with delivery facilities.
- Aaganwadi workers help them in immunization and implementation of national programmes, so the 12th pass Aaganwadi workers after receiving training should be linked to the concerned sub-centre.

Mitanin Recommendations about AYUSH

- First aid kit of Mitanins should contain allopathic and AYUSH medicines and have regular supply from district Ayurved office.
- They should receive training about the use of AYUSH and Allopathic drugs.
- Medicine supply for children especially syrups should be more.
- ANMs do not allow them to take cases to hospital for delivery and when they go to hospital do not treat them properly. Government should look in the matter.
- Training demand from most of the Mitanins about training in AYUSH and Home Remedies.
- The booklet *"Jadi Buti Lae Karo Ilaj"* is very useful.
- More training related to the use of home remedies with medicinal plants in the neighbourhood.
- Identification of medicinal plants and their local names.
- There should be posters, brochures about AYUSH available to her for explaining to community people.
- Mitanin should be linked to Ayurved dispensaries. Appointment of Mitanins should be formalised with cultural community rituals.
- There should be exposure visits to AYUSH institutions.
- Good work of Mitanins should be acknowledged and they should get cash incentives for that.
- Roles and responsibilities of Mitanins to be clearly sorted out.
- Mobilizing the potentials of 60,000 Mitanins to provide health services in hamlets and villages is a challenging task in Chhattisgarh.

Stakeholder Concerns and Remedies

Himachal Pradesh

- Shortage of doctors.
- Establishing Sub-centres under Ayurved Health Centres for expansion of AYUSH services.
- Co-location or coordination of paramedical staff under the leadership of AYUSH doctor.
- Strengths of AYUSH to be utilized for National Programmes.
- Maternity services in AYUSH hospitals to be planned.
- MIS of AYUSH to be systematically developed and used for publication of AYUSH contributions in health delivery of the State/country.
- Strengths of AYUSH in *Panchkarma Chikitsa* and geriatric care with *Rasayan Chikitsa* to be publicized and made widely available. School Health programme to impart AYUSH based health education.
- AYUSH training packages for CME of doctors, paramedics, AWWs, *Dais* to be developed.
- Developing health education material through AYUSH bureau for different categories of people.
- Cross referrals within AYUSH and with Allopathy system to be documented and publicized.
- AYUSH nursing college and AYUSH pharmacy colleges to be started.
- Demand for 10 bedded AYUSH hospital at Subdivision level, with maternity ward.
- Documentation of home remedies and linking with professional AYUSH training.

Chhattisgarh

- Strengthening of Mitanin programme by:
  - (a) Induction of Mitanin through traditional ritual in health system.
  - (b) Training of Mitanins in AYUSH.
  - (c) Supply of AYUSH kits through AYUSH Department.
- Training needs.

(a) Baiga training for 2 weeks.
(b) AYUSH training for *Dais*.
(c) Mitanin training in AYUSH.

- AYUSH dispensary to have doctor's residence.
- Under utilized AYUSH doctors to coordinate Ayurved and Godgrahita gram.
- ANM-Mitanin-AWW and primary school collocation and coordination.
- Cross referrals to be made mandatory at co-location sites.
- Providing transport to DAO for monitoring.
- RCH a nodal programme for AYUSH.
- Problem of coordination between AYUSH and Health at district level.
- Mid Day meal and Anganwadi food supplement should follow AYUSH guidelines.
- Drug packings to be attractive and quality check of drugs by accreditated laboratory.

Madhya Pradesh

- Inadequate Awareness campaigns about AYUSH.
- Health camps of AYUSH systems.
- Need for AYUSH training and training material for paramedics, like—ASHA, AWW, ANM, Herbalist.
- ASHA to be under AYUSH department.
- Co-location to be at PHC, Sub-centre and AWW level.
- Co-location site for AYUSH units in District Hospitals should be in the frontage and not backyard.
- *Infrastructure*: Own buildings are necessary as 95 per cent are currently rented. Residence for Medical Officers was in demand.
- Quality of drugs questionable. Supply doesn't match with demand.
- Plantation of medicinal plants on common village land should be encouraged.
- Food supplements in Anganwadi to be according to AYUSH guidelines.
- Anganwadis to have AYUSH medicine kits.
- Availability of vehicle at district office to supervise dispensaries.
- Pharmacists salary should be from NRHM.

Maharashtra

- Head of the State for AYUSH should be a public health person of Commissioner or Director General level.
- From district to PHC level AYUSH is integrated with Allopathy system with DHO as head of AYUSH dispensaries.
- Head of AYUSH at district should be either DAO or Additional DHO for AYUSH.
- Co-location should be of doctors with assured AYUSH drug supply.
- Practice of AYUSH at PHC needs modification, with assured supply of AYUSH drug.
- AYUSH dispensaries should be increased. Some sub-centres can be upgraded to AYUSH dispensaries by posting AYUSH doctor and supply of medicines.
- All PHCs are not supplied with AYUSH medicine kits. Due to frequent transfers of MOs, there is a mismatch between AYUSH drug availability and availability of AYUSH MO. AYUSH MOs do not get same respect as allopaths and are loaded with administrative work.
- Allopathic doctors vastly ignorant about AYUSH systems and their benefits. CME is needed for both.
- Role of AYUSH in national programmes should be studied and utilized.
- Specialized training in *Panchkarma* methods and *Kshar-sutra* to be given to AYUSH MOs.
- Different modules of training for different categories of workers like pharmacists, ASHA, AWW, *Dai*, Herbalists, Mahila Mandals etc. need to be developed.
- ASHA, AWW, and ANM should have AYUSH drug kits.
- *Dai* hut in hamlets, for institutional delivery by *dai* with assistance from ANM and AYUSH doctor.
- AYUSH based supplementary food supply in Anaganwadis.
- Medicinal plant nurseries in tribal Ashram schools where land is available and in village or forest lands of tribal areas.
- Courses of AYUSH pharmacy and AYUSH based hospital and public health nursing to be developed.

- AYUSH health education material to be developed and disseminated.
- Coordination of Vaidu (Herbalist), reputed clinician and AYUSH college with competent faculty is ideal for mainstreaming.

People represented by CBO, like Mahila Mandal, SHGs, Youth groups and by PRI are not taken as stakeholders. There is no dialogue with the people in any form on health issues. There is 50 per cent reservation for women representatives in PRI, the women could be given more authority and financial powers in regard to health issues. Anganwadi, ASHA, sub-centres could be under the control of Gram Panchayat/Garm Sabha. Experiments of putting medicine kit of Allopathic and Ayurvedic drugs in every hamlet with a volunteer like ASHA has proved to be very useful to the people. Para-medical staff has to be given more orientation and authority with their social audit done by Gram Panchayat since they enter the village homes, and not the doctors. AYUSH gram as recommended in Twelfth Five Year Plan be introduced to be monitored by PRI and CBO under the technical guidance of a NGO, if necessary.

8

EPILOGUE

Mainstreaming and Integration

AYUSH systems of Medicine have been a part of Indian Culture with each system more popular in different regions due to historical, linguistic and ecological reasons. Although homoeopathy is not of Indian origin, it has been more popular in Bengal. Currently homoeopathy has become more popular due to easy administration of therapy particularly in respect of children. During British rule, patriotic feelings about being anti-British drew some people closer to Germany, for training in Germany in preference to Britain and preferring coffee instead of tea from the British owned tea companies. Tibetan medicine has been accorded national accreditation since Dalai Lama made India his home. People have been following these plural systems according to their own genius in health care at the family, kin-group and village level. There have been traditional therapists in all these medical systems. For common ailments, people have been following a mix of home remedies and local referrals with professional knowledge of herbs.

Since, the Governments have owned the responsibility of providing health care to the people, institutionalization of public sector in health has been steadily increasing in all medical systems. In the public domain, there is an element of accountability in terms of public expenditure and measurable benefits to the people. Since medical systems are not natural sciences but applied sciences, each system through experience is endowed with particular strengths in addressing the preventive, promotive and curative aspects of health.

Although the community health institutionalization in public sector has been propagated in plural medical systems, it is desirable to organize the health care delivery in such a way as for the people to have the benefits of the strengths of all systems. It is necessary to make the systems accessible and affordable to all the people at least for primary health care. The actors in health care delivery at village level are of two types: (1) Para-medical personnel, (2) Local healers and *Dais* who possess indigenous knowledge about health care, as members of the community.

There has always been a desire in governance of health care to integrate all these systems and optimally utilize the knowledge and skills of para-professionals and professionals. These ideal wishes could not be structured in an integrated system despite several expert committees making useful recommendations. The main sociological reason for the gap between the desirable and the actual has been due to lack of reliable quantitative and qualitative data about the utilization of medical systems as home traditions and the utilization from the market sources. It was, therefore, conceived to collect the data on an all India basis on these issues. Through initiatives from the Department of AYUSH, Government of India, the two institutions, viz. The Maharashtra Association of Anthropological Sciences (MAAS) and Society for Economic Development and Environmental Management (SEDEM) were asked to undertake studies in five States. Since, the NRHM had been introduced with full steam, the National Health Systems Resource Centre (NHSRC) volunteered to study the ground reality in 18 States with the concurrence of the Department of AYUSH. SEDEM report on Rajasthan and NHSRC report about 18 States have been compounded with studies of 4 States by MAAS in this book.

Thus, an attempt has been made to present the ground situation of AYUSH in Community Health for 23 States of India, which could be generalized as getting the reality about rural India. Although the methodological focus in SEDEM and NHSRC has been of a quantitative nature and that by MAAS, more qualitative in nature, the total picture emerging for AYUSH utilization in India has been remarkably uniform. This also qualifies the methodological rigour and scientific dedication of all the studies.

Dr. Shailaja Chandra has addressed this issue in her book "*Status of Indian Medicine and Folk Healing*", Part II, by giving a resume of several surveys such as by NCAER, NFHS-2, ICMR, NSSO, CCRAS etc. (2013, 6-13). It, however, appears that several of these surveys have been health care institution based or from providers perspectives. Utilization has been computed in terms of expenditure of health care. It is difficult to compute utilization of AYUSH in respect of home remedies for common ailments, for preventive and promotive traditional patterns for mother and child health and where the services of local herbalist (*Baiga, Vaidu*) or *Dai* have been utilized and payments made in kind rather than in cash.

The studies by MAAS have been carried out with an anthropological methodology of emic approach at micro level, to look at issues from peoples' perspectives and not only patient centred. It appears, CCRAS and CCRUM have documented about 5000 folklore, ethno-medical claims made by tribal people, including ethno-medical practices, use of medical plants etc. to treat a wide ranging conditions such as common cold, cough, fever, vomiting, skin diseases, digestive problems, reproductive and child health problems, wounds, bone setting etc. (Shailaja Chandra, 2013: 10-11).

Dr. Shailaja Chandra's two volumes if read concurrently with the reports by NHSRC, MAAS and SEDEM provide holistic resume of AYUSH Public Health in India. Dr. Chandra's book deals with comprehensive issues about AYUSH including Pharmacy and Education.

Discussion

The two most often repeated terms about AYUSH during the last decade have been Mainstreaming and Integration. Mainstreaming and Integration with what or with whom? What is the Mainstream? These terms are also used about the marginalized groups such as ST, SC and other groups referred as socially and economically backward. These groups are expected to join the mainstream for their development. The principle of equity in the Constitution is invoked for their inclusive growth. Looking into the history of India and other traditional civilizations/countries which were colonized by the European powers, the traditional health care systems which were the aspects of their respective cultures got marginalized.

Now, that the attempts are being made to revitalize these systems which have stood the test of time with a separate AYUSH Ministry, a distinct National Policy and parallel health care delivery system, it also becomes obvious that at some point of time, there has to be one National Health Policy in one Nation-State and the people should get their right to access the best of all systems of medicine.

For the first time, new focal areas such as AYUSH in Public Health and Local Health Traditions were subjected to scrutiny by forming working groups by the Steering Committee on AYUSH in the Eleventh Five Year Plan. It was believed that these dimensions would serve to enhance the social and community outreach of AYUSH in the Eleventh and Twelfth Five Year Plans.

The Steering Committee advocated a two-tiered research framework for AYUSH. First tier referred to the generation of 'ocean of knowledge' over the centuries as indigenous knowledge systems having their own distinct foundations, principles, world views, philosophical frameworks, theories of health and disease, therapies and concepts. It was necessary to conserve and revitalize these traditional knowledge systems.

Second tier refers to global communicability of the capabilities of AYUSH in dealing with contemporary problems of health care. Thus the standardization of drugs according to modern scientific parameters that are internationally accepted, and path-breaking health concepts and therapies related to pharmaco-genomics, drug delivery methods, human physiology, mental health, immunity, management of systemic disorders, geriatrics, maternity care and so on require inter-cultural and trans-disciplinary research.

From the anthropological perspective, it would help to revisit some observations of the report of sub-group on Public Health for the Eleventh Five Year Plan, since, the author of this book was the Chairman of the sub-group.

"The Task Force Report of Mainstreaming of AYUSH in National Health Care admirably brings out the relevant issues and recommendations for modifications in the present system while advocating functional integration of all plural medical systems in India, at all levels.

Ideally, integration should be manifested in the integrated National Health Policy and the integrated NRHM document without special treatment of mention of AYUSH under point no. 12. Distinct National Policy and Programmes of AYUSH, creation of a separate department of ISMH in 1995 and the vast infrastructure of AYUSH is an acknowledgment of the empirical realities created for the use of AYUSH for health care of the people, in the public sector, the position which AYUSH should have enjoyed as health aspect of Indian culture.

However, mere deployment of AYUSH personnel and medicines in the existing (Public Health) PHC and referral system based on modern medicine geared to western knowledge about health and disease management and the markets flooded by modern pharmaceuticals, would not lead to functional integration. These systems are headed by modern health professionals at all levels who are ignorant about AYUSH and brand it as inferior or quackery or placebo. The Public Health Programmes are targeted for global comparisons and solutions emanating at global levels. Can AYUSH contribute to health assessed in terms of its export value and promoted accordingly?"

Why AYUSH?

"The health aspect of Indian Culture and Society, historically evolved and used by the people was without external support and with the use of local health practices, traditions, indigenous knowledge and wisdom. Parts of AYUSH are expressed as great tradition in ancient books like Charak and Sushrut which evolved by conceptualizing the folk and little traditions of the common people based on empirical experience. The sustainability of AYUSH can be increased by promoting the interaction of Great and Little Traditions and through reinterpretations to suit the needs of modern times and by upscaling with the use of modern science and technology. Uniform standardised research methodology of AYUSH, not necessarily based on modern medicine, need to be evolved and systematic documentation need to be promoted."

Desirable Action towards Integration for the Health of the People

Deficiencies which need correction

(a) Number of personnel with AYUSH degrees or employed in PHCs are not the indicators of the role of AYUSH in Public Health. They work in the Allopathic system of health care delivery. In private practice also they profess and widely practice Allopathy.

(b) Public Health System of health care delivery is in the domain of modern medicine in terms of PHC and referrals up to national level. Directors of Health are Allopaths guided by targeted Nationlal Programmes.
(c) No linkage with traditional local healers with indigenous knowledge and practice.
(d) No IEC as per AYUSH in Public Health.
(e) No insurance coverage to AYUSH.
(f) No bank credit available for AYUSH institutions in the private sector.
(g) No AYUSH inputs in national programmes such as HIV/ AIDS, TB, Malaria, or at CGHS HQ or in tertiary care.

"Indian Culture has inbuilt sustainability and coping mechanisms managed by lay people in their homes and with the help of traditional healers who abound in indigenous knowledge and wisdom. It needs to be systematically studied and through constant reinterpretation, up-scaled with the use of modern science and technology, which is neither the monopoly nor creation of modern medicine. Pluralistic model will work in an integrated fashion on the same principle of unity in diversity which has to ensure mutual respect and understanding of each others' strengths, and by providing equal opportunities for all systems to develop along their philosophical genesis, experience, conceptualization and by further upscaling with the use of modern diagnostic methods of measurement of normality." (Steering Committee on AYUSH: Working Group on Public Health, 2006).

The basic issue appears to be that during discussions, surveys and recommendations, we seem to forget the public in public health or community in community health. Primary health care has been in the domain of communities with the limitations of mortality-fertility striking a balance, as reflected in pre-Independence census reports. Despite rich great traditions of health care. Primary Health Care worked well and continues to work well with management of common ailments at the household or community level. However, there have been problems of malnutrition, food security, possibly due to state controls over production processes from land and forest. There has been environmental degradation by way of pollution due to industrialization-urbanization.

Epidemics could not be controlled by traditional therapies. Modern science through immunization, antibiotics or MDT could control epidemics and mortality. Modern science and technologies could also develop green and white revolution as also methods of contraception. This led to changing emphasis from health care to health care delivery increasing the centralized authority and administration. Community contact or participation which was lost during colonial rule had to be revived with emphasis on rural development through community development movement. Disease control programmes had to be centrally administered with operational issues about supply chain of drugs, compliance leading to drug resistance etc.

It is a universally accepted human value to minimize Neonatal, Infant and Maternal mortality since the knowledge exists to do so. All these require close contact of the community with health care workers of plural medical systems which do not function in an integrated way, since they are never trained to do so, having no knowledge of plural systems.

All reports and actions in the area of health care delivery, primary, secondary and tertiary care suggest bureaucratic solutions without any dialogue or role for the community. Paramedics are close to the community in their cultural life style and by way of delivery of health care. However, the discussion about adequacy of medical personnel revolves around the ratio of doctors to population, never it is ratio of para-medics who enter the rural homes, to population coverage. Schemes like institutional delivery without equipping the health facilities are heading to exterminate the time tested institution of TBA (*Dai*). In U.K. hospitals, deliveries are conducted by midwives, not by doctors. We need more institutions for training of paramedics than of doctors. What do the doctors from AYUSH systems do in private practice or in the PHC, without supply of AYUSH medicine, under the supervision of Allopathic DHO and Director of Health in several States? The Eleventh Plan recommendation to appoint Commissioners of AYUSH from Civil Services on ICDS model was implemented in some States but not the appointment of Joint DHO or Additional DHO from AYUSH stream. Why these discrepancies in decision making in favour of Civil Services only to the exclusion of AYUSH supervision at district level?

In all health reform reports, there is no mention about the role of PRI or CBOs like Mahila Mandal or SHGs. The 73rd Amendment of the Constitution is expected to provide more powers to PRI and gram sabha with moves to provide untied funds at the discretion of the Gram Panchayat. This has already been implemented in some States for tribal panchayats. There is no mention about the monitoring of Anganwadi or sub-centre by the Gram Panchayat.

Accountability and reporting is always upwards in hierarchical bureaucracy. Never, it is downwards to the people in a hamlet or a village. Planning and implementation about primary health care has to start at the hamlet and village level, for without community involvement, the neonatal and infant mortality, maternal mortality and malnourishment cannot be controlled. Micro-planning is the answer for several ills. AYUSH training about standardized home remedies, nutrition, maternity practices, child rearing can be provided to all those who are willing to volunteer in a village. This will improve the referrals for risk cases and proper monitoring and demands of health rights. The cooking and supply of nutritious supplementary food in Anganwadi or midday meals in schools from AYUSH standpoint are the natural activities which PRIs or CBOs can manage. NGOs could provide the expertise to do so. In all these micro-level orientations and implementation, it would be desirable to utilize the experiences of *Dai*, local herbalist and knowledgeable senior citizens. Keeping them aside and providing orientation through bookish knowledge will amount to breach of trust with those whose services people use, since they are available and accessible all the time unlike the employees who are hardly available at their place of work, when needed.

Knowledge becomes a part of culture, i.e. becomes sustainable if the results are experienced by the people more frequently which is possible through the process of confidence building and capacity building. Therapeutics, food, herbs, nutritious diets are the soft aspects of health culture and are acceptable with visible results. Cause-effect relationship which could be in the area of visibility such as mosquito causing malaria or in the belief system such as sin, immoral behaviour, wrath of gods or spirits etc. are in the realm of hard aspects of health culture which could be rational or non-rational. People do not accept germ theory easily since they have an inquiry as to why somebody gets afflicted and others do not? The concept of immunity is not explainable which would satisfy the common mind. The AYSUH argument that AYUSH strengthens the immunity to fight the affliction has been seen to be acceptable to common people since several herbs are also used in cooking or in home remedies with this understanding. People continue to follow these principles and practices to enhance the immunity of neonates and infants with the use traditional herbs.

Common people think about the healthy elderly and reflect on reasons for it. One of the reasons assigned for morbidity and ill-health in the present is attributed to adulteration of food items and use of chemical fertilizers and pesticides. During field interviews, people asked as to how could they live a healthy life style while these issues were beyond their control. Integration could only refer to the conditions which would facilitate access to plural therapy with full knowledge among the health workers and the people about the relative strengths of plural systems of medicine.

Integration is not possible unless it is brought in the curricula of para-medical and medical training. We have to decide our priorities. Is it primary health care to start with the base of the pyramid going towards the cone of referrals or are we addressing ourselves to super-speciality hospitals of the global standards, percolating down to health care of common people at the hands of sub-standard personnel who could buy entrance to private medical institutions by paying huge capitation fees. These private facilities work on unnecessary diagnostic referrals to get the kick backs. A UNFPA study in which the author was involved to study the high degree of female foeticide linked to widespread use of sonography in a sugar cane rich Kolhapur district in Maharashtra, revealed ANMs getting kick-backs for referring pregnant women for sonography.

Paradoxically, in the Western World, people are attracted to Asian Medical Systems as alternative or complementary systems, tired of iatrogenic effects of scientifically developed and tested modern drugs. They have embraced yoga and undertake medical tourism for Kerala therapy or *Panchkarma*. They also prefer Indian hospitals since they are cheap and of good quality in medical care and human care.

Our priority is to address the MDG which is possible by involving the community at the hamlet level by integrating the indigenous knowledge of the people (ethno-medicine) with the institutional mechanisms created by line departments by operationalizing and people monitored convergence at the micro-level.

AYUSH and Ethnomedicine

The Task force report and XIth Plan Steering Committee report, on AYUSH in Public Health, could form the anchor for the present anthropological studies.

Anthropology as holistic study of Man and his works, respects all cultures, and all plural systems of health and medicine, since they satisfy the basic needs of respective societies. History and geography of India has bestowed us with plural systems, which we have a responsibility, to put to use for people's health and ill-health requirements.

Holistic health is manifested in body-mind-soul interaction and equilibrium, with food, plant and animal life, including micro-organisms and expressed in terms of *Vata, Pitta, Kapha* and *Sattva, Rajas, Tamas* or *Mizaj, Yin-Yang* or four humors of Hippocrates. Since Man and his culture and society is evolved, the medical systems have also evolved. Since, they all function concurrently to meet the needs of people, it means, medical sciences are not perfect sciences, but applied sciences with their respective strengths.

Why are we promoting AYUSH? We promote AYUSH because lay people, particularly in the villages are already following the principles and practices of AYUSH as a part of culture. They are using food as medicine, kitchen condiments as medicinal decoctions, plants and herbs, which are mentioned in AYUSH classics as of medicinal value. There are local indigenous herbalist professionals who treat people. They also supply herbal material to AYUSH professionals, and pharmaceutical industry. What people follow in their homes are the little or local traditions and what is given in the classic texts are the great traditions of the same health care phenomena. Only that lay people do not use the terminology of great tradition. They do not recite *samhita*. People live their cultures without saying Indian or Marathi or Bengali or some other regional or sub-regional culture. Similarly, people have their concepts of body-mind-environment and use products for health, but do not generalize the terms like Ayurved, Unani, Siddha, Chinese etc. These are given terms by the literati who structure and organize formal, great traditions.

That is why, Jawaharlal Nehru has advocated the approach of change or development, along the lines of cultural practices and values, to make the change acceptable and sustainable.

MAAS has studied the ground realities of Ethno-medicine in four States in peoples' sector visiting several families in the villages, talking to doctors, ANMs, Mitanins, ASHA, AWW, pharmacist, chemists, *dais*, local herbalists and health administrators. We also had combined meetings of the stakeholders as equal partners, discussing health issues keeping aside the professional interests and formal designations. We had FGD with Mahila Mandals and discussions at Panchayat level. The perspective of the study has been from receivers or beneficiaries angle and not from provider's angle who claim to operationalise health care delivery.

State governments' response in personal meetings has been very positive, with the remarks, that the study was intended to help the State administration in the promotion of AYUSH. Research assistants stayed in the villages with the people, for about three months and visited several households, *dai*, herbalists, ASHA, ANM and AWW as also PHC, AHC etc. From anthropological methodology, health ethnography has been attempted by the research assistants 'going native' to collect the data through the spectacles of the people.

We have tried to get response from all sectors of population and health care workers from the informal, indigenous, para-professional and professional sectors. National health programmes are implemented by the paramedics on ground. The AWW is linked with both health and education although the anganwadi has a distinct institutional set up, but so vital for mother, children and adolescent health. AWW is engaged in health work, without much of formal training in health and none about AYUSH. Primary health care approach in Health For All of WHO requires inter-sectoral coordination. The convergence of the work of all paramedics under AYUSH which is a holistic concept is desirable to reach to MDG. For short term gains, vertical disease control programmes were launched to merge them subsequently in horizontal PHC system.

People's sector basically at the household level are being presented as home remedies for treatment of common ailments, the herbs being used from kitchen and in the neighbourhood. The products are a combination of herbs, or herbs and food products, accepting food as medicine, which is also prescribed in AYUSH texts. A retired ANM in H.P. remarked, "Our Kitchen is our home dispensary". Herbs also come from backyard, village surroundings and forest, particularly in tribal belts. It has been observed in Chennai high profile locality, women collecting Neem flowers in the courtyard to use in Rasam, and the apartment building hedge that of Adulsa. A lady selling leafy vegetables shouts to sell Brahmi leaves for invigorating memory.

One of our fisher folk student from Kerala listed all home medicine from different varieties of fish. But there is a need for more multi-centric studies on fish ethno-medicine, among the fisher-folk communities and those who are traditional fish eaters all over the world.

I had interviewed village women in Vallabhagarh area on the outskirt of Delhi which is under AIIMS internship training programme with a rural hospital, and was surprised that they classified diarrhoea by colour of the stools associating different causes and treatment, as per their classification.

The studies have indicated that in rural and tribal areas, after the first line of defence from home remedies, next referral is the local herbalist, who uses medicinal herbs from the nearby forest. The third referral is the subcentre ANM and further up the Ayurvedic dispensary or PHC depending upon the nature of ailment and accessibility.

The paramedics, ANM, ASHA, AWW also follows the same route of referral services for themselves and their families. In many cases, ANM, AWW bypass the local herbalist, unless he is a known specialist for some specific ailment. ASHA, however, consults herbalist like other village women. Mitanin (ASHA) as a member of the local community in Chhattisgarh has close links with the herbalist, Baiga, who supplies herbs on demand.

People's sector as shown by the qualitative studies particularly in mother and child health is strong following health care practices, rooted in culture. NHSRC studies have reported 'baby immunity' as a condition where promotive and preventive role of AYUSH was resorted to (2010: 135).

Even the allopathic gynaecologists and paediatricians, apart from other lady doctors and technocrats, follow the health care practices in their personal motherhood as prescribed by their mothers or mothers-in-law which are actually rooted in the great tradition or classic texts of AUS.

Universal practices about medicated oil massage, special food preparations for lactation and recovery of health, and early breast feeding, citing the example of cow and calf coming together, as early as possible, are widely followed. Even the earthworm decoctions in some form are common in Maharashtra and Madhya Pradesh for improving lactation.

It needs to be noted that *Dai* support is available in post delivery period for a week or so, usually taken over by the barber's wife in Madhya Pradesh. On the contrary, midwife in an Ayurvedic dispensary functions like an attendant, whose post is recommended to be phased out. So called institutional deliveries linked with incentives to be shared by health workers is negating the centuries old services delivered by *Dai*, who would like to get more skills and knowledge about birthing practices.

Treatment by Baiga of Chhattisgarh and Vaidu of Maharashtra

The roles of traditional *Dai* and herbalists, who are called *Vaidu* in Maharashtra and *Baiga* in Chhattisgarh are very important. The herbalist are using fresh material from the nearby forests in the form of roots, leaves, flowers, tubers and bark. In Chhattisgarh, Baiga are using about 200 herbs for treatment and health care. In Maharashtra, MAAS provided training to 276 tribal herbalists for processing of herbs into medicine, such as *Bala* oil, *Shatavari Kalp, Kudaghanwati, Gandharva Haritki, Krimighnavati* etc. and provided them with utensils to continue the work, as a project on practicing anthropology focusing on malnutrition.

The women trainers from Dr. Arole's Jamkhed provided *Dai* training about birthing practices, infant care and use of herbal material for common ailments to 383 traditional *dais* and other women volunteers at the 9 sites. For institutional delivery at the local level, some *Dai* huts were constructed by the community in their style, in the village of the *Dai* who has been in demand, providing a clean, sanitary, familiar place in the same village for the woman in labour, which was accessible to family members.

Since the project has been about malnutrition of tribal children, they were provided pre-cooked, ready to eat Sattu of roasted wheat and Bengal gram for the age group 6 months to 2 years. For the lactating women, *Sattu* fortified by Shatavari, Ashwaganda, Pipli and Jyesthamadh, was provided with very good results. Why can't the anganwadi supplementary food and mid-day-meal be made according to AYUSH principles?

Administrative Issues: Integration

Himachal Pradesh is headed by Director from Civil Services and Madhya Pradesh, by Commissioner from Civil Services. Chhattisgarh is headed by Director while Maharashtra Director is supervising AYUSH Medical Education only. At the central level itself, ISMH was under an Allopath, Director General of Health Services until a new department was established in 1995, rechristioned as AYUSH in 2003. NHSRC report has provided the variable picture of administrative structure in 18 States. Either DHO from Allopathic stream is supervising all health care delivery in a district or there is a parallel authority of DAO, the two authorities right up to Directors levels not converging in any form (2010: 98-101).

AYUSH doctors have been most vocal about their marginalized status in Health System due to poor infrastructure by way of poor state of buildings, lack of furniture in dispensaries, no transport available even to DAO for monitoring, and poor instrumentation. There are hardly any promotional channels, and there is wide disparity in pay scales with allopaths. They complain that even sub-centres have better maintenance grants than the AYUSH dispensaries. Hired transport for district authority does not appear to be a functioning solution. Ayurvedic dispensaries are hardly visited by the district authorities which could result into widespread Allopathic private practice by AYUSH doctors and unrealistic statistics about OPD attendance. There is demand for pathological laboratory instrumentation and for processing of herbs. Private pathology labs in Chhattisgarh which do not go beyond blood and urine analysis, are having good private practice prescribing plural therapeutic drugs and also functioning as chemists.

However, some retired or experienced paramedics are also having good private practice, labeling themselves as AYUSH dispensary. They are spoiling the image of AYUSH. Besides there are mobile clinics in tents run by rural clad quacks who profess themselves as Ayurved trained persons and mostly practice about infertility. Some experienced herbalists have established clinics, practicing herbal medicine combining with some *Panchakarma* facilities. In Maharashtra, in some tribal blocks there are such specialist centres run by *Vaidu* mostly giving relief from paralysis. The clinics are visited by affluent from the metro cities in cars.

One striking gap is the very poor MIS AYUSH system. It is not clear as to how and where it gets coordinated with the health MIS of the district or State. Similarly, the absence of IEC institution for AYUSH, results in lack of IEC material at various levels—in schools, public institutions, media, at mass level. AYUSH is now creeping into cosmetic industry as appears from advertisement of multi nationals. CCR-AUS have produced some IEC material seen at exhibitions of *Arogya,* not yet reached the villages or tehsil places.

The ignorance of Allopathic doctors about AYUSH is colossal, although some of them prescribe branded ayurvedic products, without knowing they are Ayurvedic products.

Another striking gap is the poor indoor occupancy of AYUSH hospitals. Although majority of deliveries are at home, conducted by *Dais,* there are no maternity facilities in AYUSH hospitals. The reason advanced is lack of trained staff, no surgical back up like anesthetics, blood supply etc., as if the difficult cases cannot be referred which we claim to provide at the village level. The entire traditional health care for mother and children are the strength of AYUSH practiced in homes. However, RCH remains outside the purview of AYUSH. AYUSH doctors do perform family planning surgeries but are not trained for the ceasarians. AYUSH does not seem to be incorporating the surgical image of Susrut. *Kshar-Sutra* is, however, very popular and effective. There is a demand for *Panchkarma* clinics to give a distinct, visible identity to AYUSH, which has become famous internationally.

In Maharashtra, co-location has been projected in terms of appointment of BAMS in the PHCs where, in remote areas, MBBS are not available. WHO has commented about this induction "to think of it as no more than a possibly useful source of manpower, to increase the coverage of official health services." The question, is what does the BAMS physician do in the allopathic PHC supervised by allopathic DHO or an Allopathic Director of Health Services? It is very confusing as to what happens to infrequent ayurvedic kits in PHCs when the doctors are MBBS? They are used when the Allopathic drugs are in short supply. There is nothing like a DAO in Maharashtra and the Director of Ayurved has no public health function, but to supervise 116 AYUSH undergraduate medical institutions, the largest in number in the country in one state besides postgraduate institutions. Maharashtra has 63 Ayurvedic, 5 Unani and 48 Homoeopathy medical colleges. As homeland of homoeopathy; even West Bengal has only 13 Homoeopathy colleges. In other three State, each study district has about 70 AYUSH dispensaries supervised by DAO, while in Pune district in Maharashtra, there are 13 Ayurvedic dispensaries and 8 Primary Health Units under PHC, with unclear dual supervision by DHO and Assistant Director Ayurved incharge of a circle covering 6 districts.

Stakeholders Consultative Meetings

Meetings of health care delivery staff of paramedics and medics were held at the district or tehsil place culminating in meetings at State level. The idea was to discuss the issues about AYUSH and Public Health in a free atmosphere keeping aside one's designation and hierarchies.

The best meetings were in Himachal Pradesh where all levels of paramedic and medical staff were present along with elected representatives at block and district level. Each participant mentioned that such a meeting was held first time in their careers.

The State meeting was presided over by the Minister of Health and Ayurved, who has been an Ayurved physician. He made three important points.

1. Study team to advise about mainstreaming of home practices in health care.
2. Advising the AYUSH practitioners from AYUSH Health Centres that preventive and IEC work under their area was their job responsibility.
3. Not to compare with Allopathic system.

The District meeting at Sagar in M.P. brought out the motivation of AYUSH doctors and the Chhattisgarh meeting was attended by a pro-AYUSH retired Director of Health. Maharashtra meeting was held at Pune, attended by Joint Secretary, Public Health, Government of Maharashtra and SHSRC director besides NGO, Medical College faculty etc.

All these meetings were initiated as part of Project methodology as consultative meetings.

Some of the other important points emerged in these meetings:

(a) If we think of co-location for choice of patients, the public should be made aware about the strengths of AYUSH through IEC.
(b) Co-ordination or cross-referral be made mandatory in some form to avoid duplication.
(c) The fundamentals of all AYUSH systems should be known to all AYUSH practitioners including the allopaths. Since modern medical colleges are totally devoid of AYUSH knowledge, it can be done through CME workshops.
(d) AYUSH Day should be celebrated all over the country on a particular day by the Ministry of Health.
(e) Co-ordination at Block and District level has to be structured by way of quarterly meetings.
(f) Residence should be attached to Ayurvedic dispensaries for the doctor and staff to stay.
(g) All untrained *Dais* who demand training be trained by AYUSH department.
(h) Herbalist and *Dai* training in AYUSH for two weeks be designed with a certificate of participation issued to them.
(i) AWW be trained in nutrition education, home remedies and AYUSH way of mother and child care.
(j) NRHM should provide AYUSH kit to ASHA/Mitanin regularly.
(k) Continuous training of ASHA in AYUSH be arranged by NRHM and AYUSH, through SHSRC.
(l) Physicians and paramedics should be encouraged for AYUSH tourism to see good hospitals and programmes.

The Allopathic doctors from PHCs and CHCs were in favour of co-location particularly in single doctor PHC to ensure doctor's availability all the time. They desired AYUSH colleagues to share the responsibility of emergency medical care and medico-legal cases. They also desired CME in AYUSH to facilitate cross referrals at co-location.

It was observed that plural therapy and cross therapy has to be consciously promoted at AYUSH co-location. Ayurved and homoeopathy were not seen referring to each other, claiming cure for all problems within their respective systems. Ayurved doctors prefer to give allopathic medicine in all cases instead of referring. Allopaths also give branded Ayurved drugs as medical representatives of Ayurved pharmaceuticals approach them.

Although AYUSH doctors participate in the national programmes, this is not acknowledged in the statistical report prepared by Health Department. All the credit goes to Health Department since AYUSH department does not publish any data-set by themselves. As one civil services Director put it, "we are subordinate, junior partners, so we do not get any credit." Another retired Director of Health of the undivided Madhya Pradesh and Chhattisgarh said, he found MBBS and BAMS equally good or bad when it comes to national programmes.

In the AYUSH dispensaries, AYUSH doctors appeared under-utilized, managing the OPD only. When they are sent to PHC, they are burdened with administrative work or School Survey. School survey could be tied with AYUSH IEC which is totally absent. There has been a demand for AYUSH sub-centres attached to AYUSH dispensaries.

There could be AYUSH health camps like *Kshar-Sutra* camps in Himachal Pradesh. AYUSH becoming a nodal agency for some national programmes helps image building and developing a distinct identity for AYUSH. Chhattisgarh has floated the schemes like Ayurved gram and Godgrahita gram which could provide health work to AYUSH doctors besides OPD work. The scheme as AYUSH gram is approved by Steering Committee in XII Plan.

There have been suggestions from AYUSH for CME in emergency care. The AYUSH doctors also prescribe Allopathic medicine since the people require quick relief for some ailments to put them on work early. In cases of risk of infection such as in *Kshar-Sutra* procedure, Allopathic drugs are prescribed, which are good examples of plural therapy.

The demand for co-location at the sub-centre, Anganwadi level was more vocal from ANM. They said, sub-centres remained closed when they visited other villages. Anganwadi has been getting AYUSH medical kit about which they have no training and it is very infrequent. They also desire AYUSH training so, that they can help women and children and communicate with local herbalist. In their personal lives, they use home remedies before trying the drugs in their kit. For quick relief, everybody tries allopathic drugs. Coincidental physical co-location of one Ayurvedic dispensary with sub-centre and anganwadi in Himachal Pradesh has given very good results in offering services. We found anaemia testing by Ayurvedic doctors with ANM, in Anganwadi as an activity of Anaemia free Himachal campaign. AYUSH training although mentioned in ASHA training is missing in practice. In Chhattisgarh, in Mitanin training, information about home remedies are given which are used. That brings Mitanin in close contact with the herbalist, Baiga. AYUSH drugs are not visible in kit of ASHA or Mitanin.

Pharmacists have mentioned about the gaps in drug supplies which are centrally supplied. There is mismatch between the requirements of specific drugs and what is supplied. Pharmacist wants instruments utensils for processing of drugs in co-ordination with local herbalist. Pharmacists and doctors recommend supplies in small and attractive packings. Otherwise they have to dispense medicine in shabby loose paper wrappings. Pharmacist would like to train the herbalist in making drugs at local level. The village representatives expressed concern about the quality of some AYUSH drugs. Plantations of medicinal herbs are recommended by village people, which is also proposed in Ayurved gram concept in Chhattisgarh.

Acceptance of the cultural concept of lifelong friend, Mitanin as equivalent of ASHA, in Chhattisgarh is laudable. However, for better results Mitanin need to be initiated in the Health system following the traditional ritual or ceremony whereby they are bound to families as friends in need, for life. Mitanin is for a hamlet which is the unit of social action and not the revenue village. This reality needs to be understood in all health care delivery issues. ASHA requires, AYUSH IEC material to share with Mahila Mandals. Monthly meeting of Mitanin with villagers has been reported in the study villages. Sub-centre and Anganwadi could become the hub of women activities and the respective places used whole day if such meetings are co-ordinated by AYUSH doctor and Sarpanch or Secretary. AWW demand AYUSH training in medicines and nutrition and diets. AYUSH based diets and supplementation need to be designed according to local conditions.

Chemists kept both Allopathic and Ayurvedic drugs. If the Ayurvedic physicians prescribe, the sale of ayurvedic drugs is about 70-80 per cent, otherwise varies from 20-40 per cent even in shops closer to PHC or CHC. Some grocery shops also keep Allopathic and AYUSH drugs where there is no chemist. Ayurvedic physicians may give Allopathic drugs for quick relief but for stomach problems, throat congestion or weakness, they prescribe Ayurvedic syrups. Women after delivery purchase Ayurvedic medicine, besides traditional health care.

Summary of Findings

The findings of studies in 23 major States in India conducted by three organizations with academic rigour and spirit, about the grassroot realities of the functioning of AYUSH systems in the backdrop of NRHM, as directed by the Department of AYUSH, Government of India could be summarized as under:

NHSRC studied 18 States with a focus on systemic approach.

The major findings of the Report has been the high utilization and valid knowledge of LHT and AYUSH that are integrated part of the lives of large sections of the population across the States even in the present time. In one-third of the 18 States under study 60-90 per cent households reported utilization of AYUSH services and about one-third reported 30-60 per cent utilization in the past three months. About the medical and para-medical personnel, it is argued that the socialization in family and the community make them aware and give knowledge about LHT and AYUSH. But, their professional training and former disciplines tend to alienate them from their cultural moorings and local ecology. It appears that the O.P.D. attendance and public facilities was found to be closely associated with the quality of AYUSH services.

"In the States with poor coverage of Allopathic institutions or lack of Allopathic doctors in them, a higher coverage with co-located services may only mean a substitution of Allopaths by the AYUSH Doctors as in several PHCs in Odisha and in Jammu and Kashmir and Uttarakhand" (in Maharashtra also).

About the validation of the prescriptions of AYUSH Doctors about 80 per cent to 95 per cent prescriptions were validated by AYUSH texts, references and principles in all the States, where prescriptions were recorded. The Report have made recommendations about the planning paradigm for health care development.

Recommendations (NHSRC)

The Planning Paradigm for Health Care Development

If decentralized planning and implementation with community involvement is to be achieved in accordance with the spirit of NRHM, community needs in terms of AYUSH and LHT are required to be incorporated in planning. In fact, if the bottom-up paradigm of planning is to be adopted, then these have to be the starting point for consideration of people's health care, and 'architectural correction' of the health care system as a whole should be designed with this perspective. A framework for such an approach is outlined below:

(i) Each district must plan beginning from its epidemiological data on morbidity and mortality, and from information about the prevailing health seeking behaviours of all sections of the local people, including use of LHT, AYUSH and Allopathy. Documentation and validation of these should be an ongoing task at the district and State levels.

(ii) The documentation of health seeking behaviours should be an activity required of the AYUSH doctor at the PHC and CHC. The local traditional practitioners, the panchayat and the VHSC should be associated with the activity.

(iii) The documentation could be collated at district level as community knowledge, the traditional practitioners' practices being certified by the panchayat as locally beneficial knowledge.

(iv) Use of the LHT and AYUSH for MCH, NCDs and any other conditions found suitable must be identified and promoted for self-care, home-based care and institutional care, as appropriate. Each state should generate 'Multi-pathy' Standard Guidelines for Treatment for all health care providers (including the doctors of Allopathy and AYUSH, ANMs and ASHAs), stating the role of AYUSH and LHT in primary care and the points of cross-referral. This requires assessment of cost-effectiveness of optional regimens from home remedies to AYUSH to Allopathy at primary, secondary and tertiary levels.

(v) Campaigns initiated by the Department of AYUSH, such as for MCH in Homeopath, Geriatric services and the Kshaar Sutra for ano-rectal disorders currently being undertaken by selected stand-alone Ayurveda institutions, should be taken up at the co-located services as well.

(vi) The AYUSH graduates who receive clinical training in conducting normal deliveries could provide MCH services (including deliveries) in the stand alone institutions. They could involve the local *dais* as support in the deliveries, as well as for ANC and PNC.

(vii) The use of AYUSH and LHT in epidemic situations (as already undertaken for Chikungunya and dengue in some States) needs to be studied and incorporated into public heath practice in other States.

(viii) These steps would be given the 'mainstreaming of AYUSH' strategy its content so that it does not merely become the 'mainstreaming of AYUSH providers'.

(ix) Use of the HMIS for regular monitoring of implementation of plans and quality of services, identifying gaps and thereby strengthening inputs would then improve quality as well (NHSRC 2010: xxxvi-viii).

Rajasthan Report has widely used the anthropological terms of Little Tradition and Great Tradition giving quotes from the XI Plan Recommendations of the Planning Commission on AYUSH and Public Health. The Report (pp. 27-33) has provided data about the commonly used systems by the people in Rajasthan. In case of children, AYUSH is exclusively used in treating Fever (84%), Diarrhoea (75%), Skin Diseases (14%) and Anaemia (13%). While the same percentage for adult males is slightly less. Among the females, AYUSH is used exclusively for treating Gynaecological disorders (76%), 49 per cent for treating Fever and 37 per cent for Diarrhoea. The elderly used AYUSH more for Asthma (51%) and for treating Joint Pain (57%), 48 per cent for Fever and 44 per cent for Diarrhoea. For about 24 common ailments ranging from common cold to minor injuries, the utilization of AYUSH only varies from 93 per cent to 58 per cent by the AYUSH Doctors. The AYUSH Doctors have accepted home remedies to be effective and need to be promoted. 85 per cent AYUSH Doctors have accepted that there are no AYUSH specific components in the training of ASHA. ASHA only carry the kit provided to them and do not promote LHT for home remedies.

ASHA and AYUSH Component within NRHM

Nearly 85 per cent AYUSH doctors say that no AYUSH specific components have been included for ASHA. Responses from ASHA interviewed at Ajmer indicate that they don't promote LHT or home remedies; they simply carry the kits and dispense what they should. The user groups also confirm that ASHA do not normally recommend home remedies or promote LHT. Very few doctors responded in the affirmative that AYUSH components have been included in ASHA's training module (SEDEM, 2010: 31).

MAAS studies in four States of Himachal Pradesh, Madhya Pradesh, Chhattisgarh and Maharashtra brings out the widespread knowledge and use of home remedies for common ailments by the people. Services of local herbalists (*Baiga, Vaidu*) and *Dai* or senior ladies with *dai* experience are also widely accessed. The AYUSH system and PHC system for primary health care in the three States function as parallel rails with no convergence in sight. NRHM in terms of co-location has been functionally non-existent although the health personnel expressed the usefulness of such a system with proper orientation and CME. In Maharashtra, integration refers to employment of BAMS in the PHC system mostly in tribal belts where MBBS are not available, with a total mismatch between the postings and supplies of Ayurvedic medicine.

The para-medics are using AYUSH as members of community which they have imbibed through socialization and enculturation, but not as part of the health care delivery system. They desire AYUSH training and kits. In Chhattisgarh Mitanin programmes are fairly structured, with training modules on home remedies.

Supply of AYUSH kits to ASHA/Mitanin and AWW have been very irregular, almost getting into history.

Refreshing reference is desirable about the studies undertaken under the guidance of Ms. Shailaja Chandra, Former Secretary, Department of AYUSH, Government of India on "Status of Indian Medicine and Folk Healing", Part I and II. The Principal Investigator has made several far reaching recommendations about medical and para-medical education in the context of NRHM. The reports need to be read in original. However, the author of the current book made a review for JAIM, the abstracts of which could be quoted to summarise the recommendations."

This status report is an encyclopaedic road map for AYUSH in India with focus on issues of integration of AYUSH with modern medical therapy. The least that the Department of AYUSH could do is to appoint Expert Committees to prepare the relevant strategies and schemes for administering the recommendations given in the book on the 'comprehensive agenda' discussed in detail on the basis of field visits and widespread discussions.

We are all aware that the medical education in all systems of medicine is more treatment oriented than public health oriented. However, the therapeutic strengths of various systems are also not organized in favour of the people. There is a need to introduce AYUSH modules in MBBS curriculum and more so in the training of paramedics. In this context, the author has discussed the issues of credibility of *Panchkarma* treatment which has gained international acclaim leading to medical tourism. Similarly, the non-invasive procedure to manage and treat piles and similar disorders by *Ksharsutra* need to be promoted. The modern medical practitioners and health administrations have been found to be totally ignorant of such therapies.

NRHM tried to bring coordination between AYUSH and modern therapy by physical co-location of the clinics which has met with resistance from the modern medical health care system. In Himachal Pradesh, there are more Ayurved Health Centres (AHC), then Primary Health Centres (PHC) in close vicinity of each other. However, there is no congruence between the two. The AHC OPDs have less number of patients which the finance administration resents in view of the high emoluments paid to the doctors. However, an issue that pregnant women in the area of AHC or the children are not patients who would visit the OPD, but their health continues to be the State responsibility. AHCs need to provide that preventive and promotive care. They demand the staff like ANMs, when the solution lies in the networking of AHC and PHC. Briefly, the concept of Public Health in AYUSH sector has yet to be developed.

The author has dealt at length the issues of medical education and research in all aspects of health care. It has been advocated to institute AYUSH Chairs in medical colleges for cross disciplinary education. The ten-year integrated MBBS/MD/Ph.D. Course in integrative Medicine is advocated. AYUSH services have been recommended to be provided in all institutes under MoHFW. A joint ICMR-AYUSH body to promote interdisciplinary research has been recommended. The author who was herself Secretary of AYUSH has commented on the necessity of senior health administrators to understand the Government Policy of integration or congruence in order to make full use of strengths of AYUSH (JAIM: Vol. 4-3, July-September 2013, pp. 184-185).

In short, author has made some comprehensive recommendations for the utilization of AYUSH to occupy its proper place in health care in all aspects.

- Ayurvedic Psychiatry in Kerala need to be studied for replication.
- Reimbursement of AYUSH treatment in the Government sector on par with modern medicine, as also the insurance cover for AYUSH treatment need to be given.
- Credit facility for development of AYUSH facilities, in the private sector need to be formalized by the nationalized banks on par with modern medicine.

Shailaja Chandra has appreciated that hundreds of home remedies have been compiled by CCRAU, but "the concern is how these time honoured home and community level practices would continue to be used in the years to come despite having been in the first line of treatment for generations" (2013: 4). It is recommended to promote AYUSH based life style guidelines for RCH, adolescent health, geriatric care, mental health, non-communicable diseases, anaemia, nutrition and health promotion through holistic behavioural change packages or patterns.

Recommendations

1. Mainstreaming and Co-location

It was observed that the status of AYUSH health delivery system is different in different States and has evolved over the years in response to geographical, political and socio-economic environment of the State including biodiversity and cultural responses, traditional beliefs and practices and needs of the people. Therefore, it was realized that the operational strategies for Mainstreaming of AYUSH need to be understood for planning strategies in each state. Mainstreaming should operationally mean full utilization of the strengths of each system in health care delivery. Similarly, Co-location should ideally mean availability of these respective systems and strengths under one roof or in the neighbourhood of each other. Lay people for common ailments accept any system which gives quick relief and is accessible and affordable without bothering about choice of system.

2. *Vertical Systems* Versus *Integrated Plural Systems*

(a) *There should have been Integrated National Health Policy for India:* As there is a separate AYUSH (ISMH) policy, the vertical AYUSH system need to be functional, gradually progressing towards integration as in many disease control programmes like malaria, leprosy etc.

(b) *Government AYUSH sector at State, District and Block level:* As per the Steering Committee recommendations of having a Commissioner for AYUSH with Secretary's powers at State level, as in ICDS model, who is funded by Central Government and partly accountable to it is necessary.

In States like Maharashtra, there has to be AYUSH authority/officer at district and block level equivalent to existing health authorities as in other study States.

(c) *Ignorance about AYUSH systems and their strengths among Government health sector*: Respect to AYUSH systems in Government sector would be possible only when there is awareness about time tested strengths of AYUSH systems among the mainstream allopathy health functionaries at medical and paramedical levels. Due to this ignorance coordination in the Government health sector is the main hurdle towards Integration. The strengths of AYUSH systems are being validated by modern scientific parameters. However, laboratory based and animal experimentation based methods of validation may not be needed for AYUSH as body-mind interaction can be experienced.

This calls for properly documented clinical experiences and a good MIS system for AYUSH. It also calls for frequent updates through CME programmes at all levels. Reforms in formal medical education are necessary in all systems of medicine.

3. *Strengthening of People's Sector*

People's sector has been functioning since ancient times. Health practices of people gradually became great traditions of classical texts compiled by intellectuals like Charak, Sushruta and Vagbhat, in all the traditional Asian systems. People's sector need to be strengthened as it is organically linked with these classic texts. Ayurveda is not only herbalism, but all herbalism is based on Ayurveda and other systems.

Health care practices, work of *Dai* and herbalist are to be linked to health institutions which could be done by collocation and coordination at village and block level under the leadership of AYUSH doctors.

4. *Role of AYUSH Doctors*

AYUSH doctors have to be engaged beyond curative practice in OPD. They could coordinate Sub-centres and Anganwadis. Institutional deliveries can not be the only prime job of ASHA.

5. *Independent AYUSH Units/Institutions*

(a) State level independent AYUSH IEC unit for health education material in local language is needed.
(b) There has to be a national level nodal Institution for AYUSH public health and nursing colleges which are beyond the regulatory authority of existing Nursing Council of India.

6. Training Needs in AYUSH

(a) There is a huge demand in all the States by grassroots level workers and higher levels of health functionaries in the Government sector and people's sector like ASHA, *Dai*, Herbalists and AWW for AYUSH training which need to be managed by AYUSH department.

(b) Large number of AYUSH pharmacists are to be trained and recruited to fill the vacancies. CME for pharmacists was in demand as the existing pharmacists after their appointment are never exposed to recent advances in their speciality.

(c) CME for AYUSH doctors need to be given priority.

7. National Health Programmes with AYUSH as Nodal Agency

National health programmes under nodal initiatives of AYUSH can be developed for Mother and Child Health, Anaemia control as in Himachal Pradesh or *Kshar Sutra Chikitsa*. AYUSH institutions and PHC sub-centres have to be equipped for institutional deliveries with inputs from AYUSH trained *Dais*.

8. AYUSH and Nutrition

(a) Anganwadi as a nodal institution for supplementary food distribution need to be transformed as an ideal place for AYUSH based nutrition and diet education to the local community with linkages to Mahila Mandals and Self-help Groups.

(b) Supplementary food need to be prepared according to AYUSH principles and as per local requirements and availability of raw food grains.

(c) The supplementary food could be fortified with AYUSH drugs/herbs for different age groups of women and children. Food supplements of raw cereals given at home are totally non-functional for the purpose of health of women and children.

9. AYUSH Visibility

For image building, self-confidence and self-respect it is necessary to improve the infrastructure of buildings, electricity and water supply, telephone connections, the maintenance of clean premises, equipments and furniture, and most important the availability of trained health manpower as per the requirements. It was reported by doctors in Himachal Pradesh that the PHC sub-centres in their areas are better maintained than AHCs due to availability of maintenance grants. Some District Ayurved hospitals and Ayurved dispensaries can be developed as a model and places of medical tourism with medicinal plantations in the premises, local folk music in play with availability of attractive food outlets with AYUSH based snacks. In Kerala and Tamil Nadu such type of clinic environment attract pregnant women for institutional deliveries.

10. Implementation of Steering Committee Recommendations

For Eleventh Five Year Plan about AYUSH in public health need to be operationalised.

Two important new dimensions were added to AYUSH in the Eleventh Plan exercise, viz. (a) role of AYUSH in Public Health, and (b) revitalization of community based local health traditions. These themes were expected to enhance the community outreach of AYUSH in the Eleventh Five Year Plan, and contribute to the overall health sector goal of "reaching the unreached".

Some of the important recommendations of the Public Health Working Group have been:

- Design pilot public health programmes related to eco-system specific herbal remedies, home and community herbal gardens, clean drinking water, non-specific diarrhoeas, anaemia, MCH etc. for introduction into the National Rural Health Mission (NRHM).
- Provide systematic, institutionalized and high quality short-term training to AYUSH medical practitioners and paramedics in public health at various levels before their deputation to the primary healthcare system across the country.
- Install an AYUSH referral system at all levels from the village to the state level with equal salaries, promotional channels and supply of medicine and equipments on par with Allopathy, sharing state of the art diagnostic facilities.
- Promote a comprehensive AYUSH Maternal and Child Health Programme in select districts/tehsils/blocks.

- Support under a coordinated programme, a network of AYUSH institutes and competent NGOs to carry out epidemiological research from an AYUSH perspective in selected districts.
- Introduce pilot projects in selected districts on preventive health for school children.
- Review the Information, Education and Communication (IEC) Scheme and suggest ways in which it can be expanded and professionally managed.
- Develop AYUSH health awareness programmes and IEC materials for common people as well as for modern health professionals and paraprofessionals.
- Develop AYUSH initiatives in Water and Sanitation Programmes.

Looking Ahead

The academic need is to have more applied, practicing field social scientists, field medical anthropologists going beyond the social doctors, the professional social workers who practice social therapeutics. That would ensure research, documentation and micro-planning in partnership with the community. What is required is intervention or action research going beyond ethnography of health practices or documentation about traditional healers.

The next step would be to train AYUSH personnel in epidemiology to be able to assess the health needs and disease burden in the geographical area under their supervision. The concept of Ayurved gram initiated in Chhattisgarh has been accepted under Twelfth Five Year Plan as AYUSH gram. The epidemiological studies of *Panchkarma, Ksharsutra* therapy, adolescent health issues, reproductive and child health issues have to be undertaken at the PHC sub-centre and AHC level. One has to move from AYUSH in Community Health in Primary Health Care to AYUSH in Public Health. Unless AYUSH is incorporated in health care delivery with its strengths, it cannot take its rightful place and make significant contribution to national health policy to honour the health rights of the people of India.

Annexures

Annexure 1

Home Remedies of 4 States

Sl. No.	*Ailment*	*States*			
		Himachhal Pradesh	*Madhya Pradesh*	*Chhattisgarh*	*Maharashtra*
1	2	3	4	5	6
1.	Cough	Carom Seeds *(Ajwain)*, Fennel Seeds *(Sauph)*, Licorice *(Mulethi)*, Dry Ginger *(Adrak)*, Black Cardamom *(Elayachi)*, Honey *(Shahad)*, *Harad*, Cumin Seeds *(Jeera)*, *Vanaksha*, Holy	*Ginger (Adrak)*, Holy Basil *(Tulasi)*, *Sanjeevani Vati*, Honey *(Shahad)*, Cloves *(Laung)*, Garlic *(Lahsun)*, Peacock feather	Holy Basil *(Tulasi)*, Ginger *(Adrak)*, Piper Nigrum *(Kali Mirch)*, Dry Ginger *(Saunth)*, *Peeper*, Jaggery *(Gud)*, Eucalyptus	Ginger *(Adrak)*, Black Pepper *(Mire)*, Holy Basil *(Tulasi)*, Carom Seeds *(Ova)*, Black Chebulei *(Hirda)*, *Sitopaladi churn*, Winter cherry

1	2	3	4	5	6
		Basil *(Tulasi)*, Piper Nigrum *(Kali Mirch)*, *Mag, Makke ki gulli Geru Suhaga*	*(Morpankh)*, Turmeric powder *(Haldi)*, Jaggery *(Gud)*, Outer covering of bark of Babul tree *(Babul ki Chhal)*, *Kanji ki Chhal*, *Bokbilya*, *Bhilma*, Mango tree leaves *(Aam ka patta)*, *Panpatta*, *Lakhera*, Outer covering of bark of Pomegranate tree *(Anar ki chhal)*	leaves *(Nilgiri patti)*, Asafoetida *(Hing)*, Garlic *(Lahsun)*, Fenugreek seeds *(Methi)*, Mustard oil *(Sarason ka Tel)*, Indian Nightshade *(Bhaitkataiya)*, Turmeric powder *(Haldi)*, Milk *(Dudh)*, *Hirva Zor*, *Karil*, Clove *(Laung)*, *Kulanjal*	*(Adulsa)*, Outer covering of bark of *Babul* tree *(Babula ki sal)*, Lemon grass *(Gavati chaha)*, Pulp of Aloe vera *(Korfad gar)*, Turmeric powder *(Haladi)*, *Kapur* apply on chest, *gugula sal*, Honey *(Madhu)*, Cloves *(Lavang)*, Dry Ginger *(Saunth)*, Garlic *(Lasun)*, Fennel Seeds *(Badishep)*, Flower of Madar *(Rui fool)*, Betel leaves *(Nagveli ki pane)*

1	2	3	4	5	6
2.	Cold	Water vapour, *Sapheda*, Cumin seeds (*Jeera*), *Vanaksha*, Holy Basil *(Tulasi)*, Margosa leaves *(Neem patti)*, *Gulaj*, Turmeric *(Haldi)*, Ginger *(Adrak)*, *Jufa, nak chikadu*, Mustard oil, Garlic *(Lahsun)*, *Ratan jyot*, *Gud*, Ground nut, Coconut pulp, Dates *(Chuare)*, *Kishmish*	Holy Basil leaves *(Tulasi)*, Garlic *(Lahsun)*, Ginger *(Adrak)*, Milk *(Dhudh)*, Karench, Asafoetida, Dry Ginger, Urine of *Bachhiya*, *Mali mirch*, Cloves *(Laung)*, Black Pepper *(Peeper)*, *Babbul*, Honey, Water vapour	Water vapour, *Hara*, Honey, *Dahiman*, *Bach Kanda*	Holy Basil, Garlic, Lemon grass, Turmeric powder, Jaggery, Onion, Water vapour, *Bajra atta Ki dhuri*
3.	Fever	Dry Ginger, *Banaksha*, Fenugreek seeds *(Methi)*, Ginger *(Adrak)*, *Bakasa*, Holy Basil Leaves *(Tulasi)*, Cumin seeds *(Jeera)*, Ginger *(Adrak)*, Black Cardamom *(Elayachi)*,	Margosa leaves *(Neem)*, Cordifolia *(Gurvel)*, Leaves of Lemon plant *(Neembu patti)*, Castor leaves *(Andi patta)*, *Edulan*, Holy Basil	Stone Breaker *(Bhui Neem)*, *Gataran ki gofari*, Outer covering of bark of Mango tree *(Aam ki chhal)*, Black Pepper *(Peeper)*,	Juice of Stone Breaker *(Bhu Nimb)* leaves, Margosa *(Neem)* leaves, Indian Fumitory *(Pappada)*, *Satapa leaves*, Mint

1	2	3	4	5	6
		Black Chebulei *(Harad)*	leaves *(Tulasi)*, Dry Ginger *(Saunth)*	Long Pepper, Dry Ginger *(Saunth)*, Sugar *(Shakkar)*, Tinospora *(Guruch)*, Indian Nightshade *(Bhatkataiya)*, *Peepal ka tana*, *Chiechita*, *Margosa (Neem)*, Bail *(Bel)*	*(Pudina)* leaves juice, Dysentery Rose Bay *(Kudabi)*, Black Pepper, Cloves *(Lavang)*, Dry Ginger *(Sunth)*
4.	Constipation	Carom seeds, *Aliye ki tat*, *Triphala*, Petals of Rose flower *(Gulab ki Pankhudi)*, Black Chebulei *(Hirda)*, Belleric Myrobalan *(Behada)*, Indian Gooseberry *(Awala)*, Carom Seeds *(Ajwain)*, Juice of Lemon *(Neembu ras)*, Honey	Carom Seeds *(Ajwain)*, Black Salt *(Kala Namak)*, Guava *(Amrud)*, *Muttha*, Fenugeek seeds, Jaggery *(Gud)*, Black Chebulei, Castor oil *(Andi tel)*, Jambol *(Jamun)* Leaves, Indian	*Harra*, *Triphala*, *Chai patti*, Salt *(Namak)*, Dried Mango Powder *(Amchur)*, Carom Seeds, Clarified Butter *(Ghee)*, Aloe vera *(Ghritkumari)*, Turmeric Powder *(Haldi)*,	*Hirda*, *Amla supari* (Dry *Amla+Hing+ Jeera*), Warm milk+*Ghee*, Warm milk+*Manuka* (Black *Kishmish* or *Kharik* Dry dates, Warm water+ *Ghee*+salt

1	2	3	4	5	6
		(Shahad), Mint Leaves *(Pudiana)*, Holy Basil Leaves *(Tulasi)*	Gooseberry *(Awala)*, Lemon *(Neembu)*, Baking soda *(Khane ka soda)*, *Triphala*	Asafoetida *(Hing)*, *Peeper*, Black salt, *Gohinja*, Outer covering of bark of *Babbul*, *Dayyad (Dahiman Chhal)*, Alcohol made from Indian Butter tree *(Mahua Sharab)*, *Bagdol Ka Kand*, *Bijata ki patti*, *Lagvanti*	
5.	Vomiting	Mint *(Pundina)*, Onion *(Pyas)*, Guava leaves *(Amrud ke patten)*, *Kumbhadi Mitti*, Fennel Seeds *(Sauph)*, Fenugreek seeds *(Methi)*, Salt *(Namak)*,	Black Cardamom *(Elayachi)*, Honey *(Shahad)*, Mint *(Pudina)*, *Lakhera Mitti*, Feather of Peacock *(Mor Pankha)*, Cumin	*Davena patta*, Onion, Honey, Mint	Lemon juice *(Limbu ras)*, Salt *(Meeth)*, Sugar *(Shakkar)*, Turmeric powder *(Haladi)*, Pulp of Aloe vera

1	2	3	4	5	6
		Sugar *(Shakkar)*	seeds *(Jeera)*, Black Salt *(Kala Namak)*, Betal Nut *(Supari)*, Onion *(Pyaz)*, Jambol *(Jamun)*, Ginger *(Adrak)*		*(Korphad gar)*
6.	Jaundice	Sugar Cane juice *(Ganna Ras)*, Raddish *(Muli)*	Sugar Cane, *Kahira*, Milk, Root of Papaya plant *(Papeeta jad)*, Leaves of Radish *(Muli ke patten)*, Aloe vera *(Gvarpatha)*, Ginger (*Adrak*), Asparagus *(Satavar)*, Black Pepper *(Kali Mirch)*, Clarified Butter (*Ghee*), Sugar	Banana *(Kela)*, Raddish, Yoghurt *(Dahi)*, Mango, Outer covering of bark of Jambhol *(Jamun)* and Indian Butter tree *(Mahua ki Chhal)*, *Piri*, Leaves of Drumstick *(Munga ke patten)*, Dodder *(Amarvel)*, *Bankapas ki Chhal*, Sugar Cane juice	Stone Breaker *(Bhui Awala)*, *Tentu*, Outer covering of Bark of *Asok (Ashok Sal)*, Urine of Cow *(Gomutra)*, Lemon *(Limbu)*, Sugar *(Shakkar)*, Salt *(Namak)*, Thorn Apple *(Dhotra)*, Castor plant *(Erand)*, Tinospora *(Gulvel)*, Extract

1	2	3	4	5	6
					from Calotropis plant *(Rui cha chik)*
7.	Diarrhoea	Salt *(Namak)*, Sugar *(Shakkar)*, Fennel seeds *(Sauph)*, Clarified Butter (*Ghee*), *Katcha* Milk *(Dudh)*, Banana *(Kela)*, Almond *(Badam)*, Sugar *(Mishri)*, *Kadavi Sauph*, Fenugreek seeds *(Methi)*, Black chebulei *(Harad)*, Indian Gooseberry *(Awala)*	Bail (*Bel*), Jambol fruit *(Jamun)*, Flame of forest *(Palash)*, *Awala*, *Koha*, Outer covering of bark of Sandan *(Tinsa ki Chhal)*, Yoghurt *(Dahi)*, *Mattha*, Leaves of Tamarind *(Emali patten)*, Mint Leaves *(Pudina)*, Dry Ginger *(Sonth)*, Honey *(Shahad)*, Outer covering of bark of Mango tree,	Salt *(Namak)*, Sugar *(Shakkar)*, Lemon *(Neembu)*, *Dashman*, Tea tree leaves *(Chai patti)*, Outer covering of bark of Mango *(Aam ki chhal)*, *Dubi*, Bail *(Bel)*, *Sarai ki chhal*, Eucalyptus *(Nilgiri)*, Asparagus *(Satavar)*, Dry Ginger *(Sonth)*, Land Calotrops *(Saphed Musali)*	Drink made up from Lemon juice *(Limbu sarbat)*, *fangalyacha ras*, *Ronachi sal*, Turmeric *(Haladi)*, *Borachi sal*, *Chitrak mul*, *Murud sheng*, Aloe vera *(Korfad)*, Silk Cotton tree *(Sawar sal)*, *Kumbhai sal*, Mixture of Yoghurt and sugar *(Dahi shakkar)*, Juice of root of Periwinkle

1	2	3	4	5	6
			Silk Cotton tree *(Aam, Semar ki Chhal), Suleha, Aat,* Milk *(Dudh)*		*(Sadafulichya mulancha ras),* Sago *(Sabudana) kheer*
8.	Skin Disease	Margosa Leaves *(Neem), Meetha Soda,* Holy Basil *(Tulasi)*	Margosa *(Neem),* Cow's Urine, *(Gomutra),* Cow Dung *(Gobar),* Sulphur *(Gandhak),* Beehive *(Madhumakhi ka chhata),* Mustard Oil *(Sarson ka tel),* Thorn Apple *(Dhatura),* Holy Basil *(Tulasi), Chiraul, Ghamra,* Silk Cotton Tree *(Sem ke patten),* Camphor *(Kapur),* Coconut oil	Tomato *(Tamatar),* Margosa leaves *(Neem ki patti),* Holy Basil Leaves *(Tulasi),* Cow Dung *(Gobar), Kosam tel,* Caron Seeds *(Ajwain), Phundaraban*	Juice of leaves of Margosa *(Neem),* Vegetable gourd *(Phangala)* leaves, Extract from Calotropis plant (*Rui*), Trellis – Vine Creeper *(Utaran Vel),* Cow's Urine *(Gomutra)*

1	2	3	4	5	6
9.	Toothache	Cloves *(Laung)*, Juice of Lemon *(Neembu Ras)*, Alum *(Phitkari)*, Mustard Oil *(Sarso Ka Tel)*, Salt *(Namak)*, Carom Seeds *(Ajwain)*	Cloves *(Laung)*, Juice of Lemon *(Neembu Ras)*, Alum *(Phitkari)*, Mustard Oil *(Sarso Ka Tel)*, Salt *(Namak)*, Carom Seeds *(Ajwain)*	Indian Nightsahde *(Bhatkataiya)*, Rock Salt *(Sendha namak)*, Royal Poinciana *(Gulmohar)*, Turmeric Powder *(Haldi)*, Mustard oil *(Sarso ka tel)*	Clove (Lavang) at affected site, *Kapur* (Camphor), Common salt + Turmeric at affected tooth
10.	Headache	Dry Ginger *(Saunth)*, Carom seeds *(Ajwain)*, Mustard oil *(Sarson Ka tel)*, Fenugreek seeds *(Methi)*, Nutmeg *(Jaiphal)*, Sesame oil *(Til ka Tel)*, Ginger *(Adrak)*, Holy Basil *(Tulasi)*, Black Cardamom *(Elayachi)*, Black Pepper *(Kali*	Eucalyptus, Mustard *(Rai)*, Cloves *(Laung)*, Ginger *(Adrak)*, Sandal wood *(Chandan)*, Holy Basil *(Tulasi)*	Garlic *(Lahsun)*, Onion *(Pyaz)*, Bitter Gourd *(Karela)*, *Ghutvar*, Thorn Apple *(Dhatura)*, Eucalyptus	Indian Gooseberry *(Awala)*, Clarified butter (*Ghee*), *Hujamul*, Rock salt *(Shendeloan)*, Garlic, Lime *(Chuna)*, Roots of Lead wort *(Chitrak Mul)*

1	2	3	4	5	6
		Mirch), Fennel seeds *(Sauph)*			
11.	Injury	*Biroja*, Mustard Oil, Turmaric powder, Kerosene *(Mitti ka tel)*	*Bilja*, Black Catechu *(Kattha)*, *Gunja*, Clarified Butter *(Ghee)*, Turmeric Powder *(Haldi)*, Onion *(Pyaz)*, *Pattharchat*	*Sal*, *Goinja*, Turmeric powder *(Haldi Chuna)*, *Karanj*, Onion *(Pyaz)*, Kerosene *(Mitti Ka Tel)*, *Ratanjyot*, *Saleha*, Cow's Dung *(Gobar)*, Mustard Oil *(Sarson ka Tel)*	White mulberry *(Tendu Sal)*, Coat Button leaves *(Kambarmodi Pala)*, Turmaric powder *(Haladi)*, Outer covering of bark of *Arjun*, Lantana leaves *(Tantani Pala)*, *Raktrohida*, *Dagadi Pala*, *Awali Pala*, Aloe vera *(Korphad)*, *Khanduchhaka Pala*
12.	Bone facture	*Barne*, *Basuti*, *Gas Bel*, Milk *(Dudh)*, Raw Turmeric *(Katchi*	*Hathjudi*, *Bakari/* Cow's Milk *(Gay Dudh)*, *Chilo*, Black Catechu *(Kattha)*,	*Harsanghari*, *Koraiya*, *Amrola*, *Sarai*, *Goinja*	Wild Mango *(Ranamba)*, Cordifolia *(Gulvel)*, Devil's

1	2	3	4	5	6
		Halad)	Salt *(Namak)*, Warm Water *(Garam Pani)*		Backbone *(Hadsandhi)*

HOME REMEDIES: MAHARASHTRA SPECIFIC

Weakness	Indian Gooseberry *(Awala)*, Rock Candy *(Kadi Sakkhar)*, Clarified Butter *(Tup)*, Land Calotrops powder *(Musali Churn)*, Asparagus *(Shatavri)*, Consuming Non-Vegetarian Food *(Mansahar)*
Joint Pain	Ginger, Honey *(Madhu)*, Country Mallow *(Bala)*, Five Live chaste Tree *(Nirgundi)*, Seed of Fever Nut Tree *(Sagargota* bee*)*, *Dev Halad*, *Mirchikand*, Outer covering of bark of *Arjun*, Lead wort Root *(Chitrak Mul)*, Massage By Mustard Oil, Kerosene, Heat Treatment by Brick, Sickel senna *(Takala)*, *Melsing*, Drumstick *(Shevga)*, Leaves Juice
Pain in Lower abdomen	Ashes (*Rakh in Chulha*), Roasted Soil and Salt, Rock Salt *(Swendhav Namak)*, Carom Seeds *(Ajmoda)*, Black Salt *(Kala Namak)*, Indian Screw Tree *(Murud Sheng)*, Baking Soda *(Khanyacha Soda)*, Juice of leaves of Sorrel (*Ambadi Ras*), *Kodva*, Eucalyptus *(Nigiri)* Leaves, Dry Ginger *(Sunth)*, Dry Corriander Seeds (*Dhane*), Jaggery *(Gud)*, Seed of Fever Nut Tree *(Sagargota* Seed*)*, Common cress *(Aliv)*, Ground Nut Oil, Lantana (*Tantani)* Leaves.

Worm	Seeds of Indian Flame tree *(Palas)*, Seed of Dysentery Rose Bay *(Kuda)*, Pulp of Golden Shower Tree *(Bahava Magaj)*, *Pachar Kanda*, Seed of Drumstick *(Shevga)*, Purging Nut *(Dantimul)*, Seed of Fever Nut Tree, *Mirsing*, Juice of Bamboo Leaves, Outer Covering of Bark of Margosa tree.

Annexure 2 (a)

Home Remedies, Hamirpur District—Himachal Pradesh

RESPIRATORY SYSTEM

Cold

Sl. No.	*Home remedy Used*		*Method of Preparation*	
	Kitchen Medicine	*Medicinal Plant*	*Method of Preparation*	*Method of Use*
1	2	3	4	5
1.	Black pepper + Cumin + Cardamom + Sugar	*'Trinamool'*	Plants mentioned in kitchen medicine and/or *'Trinamool'* or only *'Trinamool'* Boiled to make decoction	Oral Intake

1	2	3	4	5
2.		Leaves of Eucalyptus tree (*'Sapheda'*)	Boiled for Vapour	Vapour-Inhalation
3.	Honey		With warm water	Oral Intake
4.	Gram flour + Semoliana Rava (*'Suji'* or *'Rawa'*) + Dry Ginger (*'Sund'*)		Crushed + water	Oral Intake
5.	Cloves + Milk		Crushed-fine powder + warm milk	Oral Intake
6.	Ginger+ Black Pepper + Holy Basil (*'Tulsi)* + *'Saunph* + *'Methi'*+ Carom Seeds (*'Ajwain'*) + Rock Salt		Plants mentioned in kitchen medicine column Boiled to make decoction	Oral Intake
7.	Cardamom+ Black Pepper + Dry Ginger (*'Sund'*) + Fennel Seeds (*'Saunph'*)	Long Pepper Long (*'Mug'*) + Wild/Sweet Violet (*'Vanaksha'*)	Plants mentioned in kitchen medicine and medicinal plants column boiled to make decoction	Oral Intake
8.	Cardamom + Black Pepper + Rock Salt + *'Tulsi'* leaves + Fennel Seeds (*'Saunph'*)	Wild/Sweet Violet (*'Vanaksha'*)	A Plants mentioned in kitchen medicine and medicinal plants column Boiled to make decoction	Oral Intake
9.	Ladies Finger Seeds (*'Bhindi'*)		Ladies Finger Seeds crushed to make powder to put in nostrils	Inhalation

Cough

Sl. No.	*Home remedy Used*		*Method of Preparation*	
	Kitchen Medicine	*Medicinal Plant*	*Method of Preparation*	*Method of Use*
1	2	3	4	5
1.	Cardamom	Long Pepper (*'Magh'*) + *'Malhari'*	Plant mentioned in kitchen medicine and medicinal plants column crushed to make fine powder mixed with honey	Oral Intake with warm water
2.	Ginger + Honey		Ginger juice + Honey Mixture	Oral Intake with warm water
3.	Honey	Wax Tree (*'Kakad singi'*)	Plant mentioned in kitchen medicine and medicinal plant column mixture	Oral Intake
4.	Cardamom		Roasted Cardamom	Oral Intake
5.	Black Pepper + Honey		Crushed fine powder of Black Pepper + Honey	Oral Intake with warm water
6.	Cardamom	Holy Basil (*'Tulsi'*)	Plant mentioned in kitchen medicine and medicinal plant column Boiled to make decoction	Oral Intake

1	2	3	4	5
7.	Black Pepper + Ginger + Fennel Seeds (*'Saunph'*)+ Fenugreek seeds (*'Methi'*) + Carom Seeds (*'Ajwain'*)	Holy Basil (*'Tulsi'*)	Plants mentioned in kitchen medicine and medicinal plant column boiled to make decoction	Oral Intake
8.	Salt	Chebulei (*'Harad'*)	Salt is applied to roasted Chebulei (*'Harad'*)	Chebulei (*'Harad'*) sucking/Chewing
9.	Cardamom (*'Badi Elayachi'*) + Honey	Long Pepper (*'Mag'*)	Pepper (*'Mag'*) and Cardamom (*'Badi Elayachi'*) crushed to make powder mixed with Honey	Oral Intake
10.	Honey + Black Pepper + Salt		Black Pepper powder mixed with salt and take with honey	Oral Intake
11.		Indian Liquorice (*'Mulbi'*)	A small piece of Indian Liquorice (*'Mulbi'*)	Oral sucking
12.	*'Kheel'* of Borax (*'Suhaga'*) + Honey		*'Kheel'* of Borax (*'Suhaga'*) is crushed and mixed with honey	Oral Intake
13.	Honey	Chebulei (*'Harad'*)	Chebulei (*'Harad'*) is roasted, crushed into a fine powder and taken with honey	Oral Intake
14.		Chebulei (*'Harad'*)	Seeds of Chebulei (*'Harad'*) are roasted	Oral sucking of roasted Harad

1	2	3	4	5
15.	Honey	Wax Tree (*'Kakad singi'*)	The seeds of Wax Tree (*'Kakadsingi'*) are burnt and the ash is mixed with honey	Oral Intake
16.		Black Malbar Nut ('Black *Vasuti'*)	The roots of black *'Vasuti'* are boiled to make decoction	Oral Intake

Congestion of Throat, Nose and Chest due to Cold

Sl. No.	*Home remedy Used*		*Method of Preparation*	
	Kitchen Medicine	*Medicinal Plant*	*Method of Preparation*	*Method of Use*
1	2	3	4	5
1.	Ginger + Cardamom + Fennel Seeds (*'Saunph'*)		Plants mentioned in kitchen medicine boiled in water to make decoction	Oral Intake
2.		Leaves of Eucalyptus (*'Sapheda'*)	Leaves of Eucalyptus boiled for Vapour	Vapour-Inhalation with warm water Oral Intake
3.	Honey			

1	2	3	4	5
4.		Sweet Violet *('Bankasha')*	Sweet Violet boiled in water to make decoction	Oral Intake
5.		Peppermint and Carom Seeds *('Ajwain')*	Peppermint and Carom Seeds boiled for Vapour	Vapour-Inhalation
6.	Black Pepper+ Clove		Powdered Black Pepper with Clove water	Oral Intake
7.	Rock Salt		Rock salt added in hot water	Gargling
8.	Cumin seeds	Sweet Violet *('Vanaksha')*+ Holy Basil *('Tulsi')* leaves + Hyssop *('Jupha')* flowers	Cumin seeds and plants mentioned in medicinal plants boiled to make decoction	Oral Intake
9.	Asafetida		Asafetida powder mixed with water	Local application on Chest
10.	Cloves + *Kattha*			Oral Intake
11.		Seeds of Dry Date *('Chuara')*		Oral sucking of seeds

Asthma

Sl. No.	Home remedy Used		Method of Preparation	
	Kitchen Medicine	*Medicinal Plant*	*Method of Preparation*	*Method of Use*
1.	Honey	Leaves of *Pipal*	Leaves of Pipal burnt and mixed with honey	Oral Intake
2.		Young leaves of Five Leave Chaste (*'Bana'*)	Boiled to make decoction	Oral Intake
3.	Honey	Flowers of Madar (*'Akk'*) + Malathisath	Equal amount of both ingredients from medicinal plant column mixed with Honey	Oral Intake
4.	Ladies Finger Seeds (*'Bhindi'*)		Crushed to make powder	Inhalation

DIGESTIVE SYSTEM

Gas

Sl. No.	*Home remedy Used*		*Method of Preparation*	
	Kitchen Medicine	*Medicinal Plant*	*Method of Preparation*	*Method of Use*
1.		Mint leaves	Chutney	Oral Intake
2.	Asafetida		Asafetida powder with water	Oral Intake
3.	Honey			With warm water. Oral Intake
4.	Carom Seeds (*'Ajwain'*) + Fenugreek Seeds (*'Methi'*) + Fennel Seeds (*'Saunph'*)		Boiled in water to make decoction	Oral Intake
5.	Rock Salt (*'Sendhav Namak'*)	Mint + Chebulei (*'Harad'*) + Belliric Myrobalan (*'Veda'*) + Indian Gooseberry (*'Awala'*)	All ingredients dried then powdered mixed with Rock Salt (*'Sendhav Namak'*)	Vapour-Inhalation
6.	Lemon		Lemon juice with water	Oral Intake
			Black salt applied on slices of Lemon	Oral Sucking

Pitta

Sl. No.	*Home remedy Used*		*Method of Preparation*	
	Kitchen Medicine	*Medicinal Plant*	*Method of Preparation*	*Method of Use*
1.	Black Salt + Black Pepper + Carom Seeds (*'Ajwayan'*)		All the ingredient mixed with Lassi	Oral Intake

Constipation

Sl. No.	*Home remedy Used*		*Method of Preparation*	
	Kitchen Medicine	*Medicinal Plant*	*Method of Preparation*	*Method of Use*
1.	Carom Seeds (*'Ajwayan'*)		Ajwain is soaked overnight Fine powder of Ajwain	Oral Intake
2.		Garcinia (*'Alia'*)	Pulp (*'Guda'*) of Garcinia (*'Alia'*) boiled in water Flesh of *'tat'* of Garcinia (*'Alia'*) boiled in water	Oral Intake
3.		Chebulei (*'Harad'*)	Chebulei (*'Harad'*) crushed taken with hot water	Oral Intake
4.	Onion	Mint	Chutney of A and B	Oral Intake
5.	Milk	White Rose	B boiled in milk	Oral Intake

Loose Motions

Sl. No.	*Home remedy Used*		*Method of Preparation*	
	Kitchen Medicine	*Medicinal Plant*	*Method of Preparation*	*Method of Use*
1.	Sugar+ Fennel Seeds (*'Saunph'*)+Fenugreek Seeds (*'Methi'*)		Fennel Seeds (*'Saunph'*) + Fenugreek Seeds (*'Methi'*) roasted together mixed with sugar	Oral Intake (2-3 tsp)
2.	Onion	Mint	A and B crushed together to extract juice	Oral Intake
3.		Leaves of Mango tree	Leaves of Mango tree crushed to extract juice	Oral Intake
4.	Rice + Pulse of Split Green Gram (*'Mung'*)		*Khichadi* of Rice + Pulse of Split Green Gram	
5.	Sugar+ Fennel Seeds (*'Saunph'*) + *Ghee*		Fennel Seeds (*'Saunph'*) roasted in *'Ghee'* and mixed with sugar	Oral Intake
6.	Palm Sugar + Almonds		Both these ingredients are crushed together to make a fine power	Oral Intake
7.	Almonds		Almonds are soaked in water and then scrubbed	Oral Intake
			Cloves are roasted mixed with sugar and scrubbed Almonds	
8.		Chebulei (*'Harad'*)	Chebulei (*'Harad'*) is scrubbed in cold water	Oral Intake
9.	Curd	*'Rasaut'*	*'Rasaut'* mixed with Curd	Oral Intake

Vomiting

Sl. No.	*Home remedy Used*		*Method of Preparation*	
	Kitchen Medicine	*Medicinal Plant*	*Method of Preparation*	*Method of Use*
1.	Onion	Mint	Onion and mint crushed together to extract juice	Oral Intake
2.		Mud of *'Kuemvja'*	Mud of *'Kuemvja'*mixed with water	Oral Intake

Indigestion

Sl. No.	*Home remedy Used*		*Method of Preparation*	
	Kitchen Medicine	*Medicinal Plant*	*Method of Preparation*	*Method of Use*
1.		Indian Gooseberry *('Awla')*	Fruit of Awala dried to make powder	Oral Intake
2.		Indian Gooseberry *('Awla')* + Belleric Myrobalan *('Behda')* + Chebulei *('Harad')*	Fine Powder of plants mentioned in medicinal plant column	Oral Intake
3.	Salt	Indian Gooseberry *('Awla')* +Belliric Myrobalan *('Veda')* + Chebulei *('Harad')* + Mint	Fine Powder of Indian Gooseberry + salt	Oral Intake

Piles

Sl. No.	*Home remedy Used*		*Method of Preparation*	
	Kitchen Medicine	*Medicinal Plant*	*Method of Preparation*	*Method of Use*
1.		Lotus plant	Stem covering of Lotus flower in water	This water is used for toilet purpose
2.		Unidentified white flower	B mixed in Semoliana Rava (*'Suji ka Halwa'*)	Oral Intake
3.		Indian Coral Tree *('Pangru')*		Oral Intake

Worms

Sl. No.	*Home remedy Used*		*Method of Preparation*	
	Kitchen Medicine	*Medicinal Plant*	*Method of Preparation*	*Method of Use*
1.	Bitter gourd *('Karela')*		Bitter gourd *('Karela')* is taken	
2.	Mustard Seeds		Mustard seeds roasted in clarified butter *'Ghee'*	Oral Intake
3.		Margosa *('Neem')* Leaves	The juice extracted by crushing Margosa *('Neem')* leaves	Oral Intake

ENT

Mouth

Soreness of Mouth

Sl. No.	*Home remedy Used*		*Method of Preparation*	
	Kitchen Medicine	*Medicinal Plant*	*Method of Preparation*	*Method of Use*
1.		*'Karkara'*	Flower of *Karkara*	*'Karkara'* flower is kept in the mouth and sucked
2.		Chirette plant *('Chiraita')*	Flower of Chirette plant *('Chiraita')*	Flower of Chirette plant *('Chiraita')* is kept on the tongue
3.	Black Catechu *('Kattha')*			Black Catechu *('Kattha')* is applied on the inside of the mouth

Mouth Ulcers

Sl. No.	*Home remedy Used*		*Method of Preparation*	
	Kitchen Medicine	*Medicinal Plant*	*Method of Preparation*	*Method of Use*
1.		Young leaves of Guava (*'Amrud'*) tree		The leaves are chewed
2.		Young leaves of Jambol (*'Jamun'*) tree		The gum from theses leaves is applied on the affected area
3.		Leaves of Sheesham ('Tali')	The leaves are sun-dried and powdered. The powder is taken along with cold water or milk	The powder is taken along with cold water or milk orally
4.		Leaves of Bael ('Bel')		The gum from theses leaves is applied on the affected area

Tooth Problems

Sl. No.	*Home remedy Used*		*Method of Preparation*	
	Kitchen Medicine	*Medicinal Plant*	*Method of Preparation*	*Method of Use*
1.	Cloves and Black Pepper			Cloves and black pepper are kept between the affected teeth
2.	Asafetida			Kept between the affected teeth
3.	Root of Lead Wart (*'Chitra'*)			The root is kept in the mouth
4.		Milk of Madar (*'Akk'*)		Applied on the affected teeth
5.	Oil (*'Rogan'*) of Almond			Applied on the affected teeth
6.	Carom Seeds (*'Ajwayan'*)			Kept between the teeth

Gum Problems

Sl. No.	Home remedy Used		Method of Preparation	
	Kitchen Medicine	*Medicinal Plant*	*Method of Preparation*	*Method of Use*
1.	Bark of Jambol (*'Jamun'*) tree	The bark is boiled in water and the decoction is used for rinsing the mouth to cure selling in gums.	The bark is boiled in water to make decoction	

EAR

Earache

Sl. No.	Home remedy Used		Method of Preparation	
	Kitchen Medicine	*Medicinal Plant*	*Method of Preparation*	*Method of Use*
1	2	3	4	5
1.	Garlic + Mustard Oil		A few cloves of garlic is added in mustard oil and heated-cooled the oil	Few drops of oil is put into the ears at night
2.	Mustard Oil	Leaves of *Madar ('Akk')*	Mustard oil is heated along with the leaves of Madar (*'Akk'*)	Few drops of oil is put into the ears at night

EYES

1	2	3	4	5
1.		Leaves of *'Durgadi'*	The juice extracted from the leaves of *'Durgadi'*	The juice put into the eyes
2.		Indian Gooseberry *('Awla')*		Oral Intake
3.	Salt + Water		A mixture of salt and water is made	The mixture put into the eyes
4.	Honey	Red sandal	Red sandal is scrubbed along with honey to make paste	Locally applied on eyes
5.		Indian Berberry *('Kasmale')*	*'Rasaut'* made from Indian Berberry *('Kasmale')*	*'Rasaut'* scrubbed applied on the eyes
6.		Sandal	Sandal is scrubbed along with water	Locally applied on eyes
7.	Carom Seeds *('Ajwain')*	Flower of *'Sultaj'* + Trailing Eclipta *('Gharmal')*	Carom Seeds and plants in medicinal plants column crushed together to make paste.	The paste applied on long leaves and these leaves tied on eye

NOSE

Nose Bleeding

Sl. No.	*Home remedy Used*		*Method of Preparation*	
	Kitchen Medicine	*Medicinal Plant*	*Method of Preparation*	*Method of Use*
1.		Leaves of Peach tree (*'Aadu'*) + *'Sheegan'*	Leaves crushed together to extract juice	2-3 drops of this juice is put into the nose
2.	Palm sugar	*'Dhaansoa'*	Palm sugar and *'Dhaansoa'* crushed together + Cold Water	2-3 drops of this juice is put into the nose
3.	Lemon		Slices of lemon crushed to make juice	2-3 drops of lemon juice is put into the nose

SKIN

Athlete's Foot

Sl. No.	*Home remedy Used*		*Method of Preparation*	
	Kitchen Medicine	*Medicinal Plant*	*Method of Preparation*	*Method of Use*
1	2	3	4	5
1.	Turmeric powder + Mustard oil		Turmeric powder mixed in mustard oil	Locally applied on the affected area
2.	Garlic + Cloves + Mustard oil		Garlic cloves added to mustard oil	Locally applied on the affected area
3.		Chebulei *('Harad')*	Chebulei *('Harad')* is crushed	Locally applied on the affected area

Pimples

1.		Margosa *('Neem')*	A spoonful of crushed Margosa *('Neem')* leaves is taken along with cold water	Oral Intake
2.	Gram Flour Besan *('Besan')* + Lemon + Milk	White Sandal	Gram Flour Besan *('Besan')* + Fine Powder of White Sandal + Lemon juice + Milk	Face pack applied locally

Boils

1	2	3	4	5
1.		Margosa *('Neem')*	A spoonful of crushed Margosa *('Neem')* leaves	Oral Intake
2.	Cloves		Crushed Cloves mixed with water to make paste	The paste applied locally on boil
3.	Stone + Mustard Oil		Stone is heated and dipped in Mustard Oil	Fomentation by stone on boil
4.	Mustard Oil + Red Gram *('Masur')*		Red Gram *('Masur')* is roasted and crushed and mixed with mustard oil	Applied locally on boil
5.	Asafetida		Paste made of asafetida and water	The paste applied locally on boil
6.		Margosa *('Neem')*	Margosa *('Neem')* leaves are dried, crushed and made into capsules	Oral Intake of capsules with cold water
7.		Copper Sulphate *('Neela-thotha')*	Crushed Copper Sulphate *('Neela-thotha')*	Applied locally on boil

1	2	3	4	5
8.		*'Phod-patta'* (name given by the villagers)	Mustard oil is applied over the leaf of *'Phod-patta'* and the leaf is heated	The leaf is then tied around the boils and left overnight. The next morning pus oozes out of the boil and the boil dries up and heals.
9.	Blue cotton cloth piece		A blue cotton cloth piece is rolled in the shape of a cigarette and burnt from the tip.	The burnt tip of the roll is used to burst the boil. This procedure is carried out by the lower caste people.

Itching

1.		Margosa *('Neem')*	Margosa *('Neem')* leaves added to drinking water	Oral Intake
2.	Turmeric Powder + Black pepper		Fine powder of Turmeric Powder + Black pepper	Oral Intake with Cold water
3.		Musk melon *('Kharbuj')*	Pulp/Juice of Musk melon	Applied over the affected area

Burning Sensation

1	2	3	4	5
1.	Cinnamon + Mustard oil		Crushed cinnamon is added to mustard oil and heated	Massage of the feet and palms
2.		Aloe Vera	Pulp of Aloe Vera mixed with cold water	Massage the hands and feet
3.		*'Chhoti-Kuare'*	*'Chhoti-Kuare'* crushed	Applied on the hands and feet

Allergy

1	2	3	4	5
1.	Black pepper + Clarified butter (*Ghee*)		Black pepper mixed with *'Ghee'*	Oral Intake

HAIR PROBLEM

Graying of Hair

1	2	3	4	5
1.		Indian Gooseberry (*'Awla'*)	Fruit of *'Awla'*/Juice of *'Awla'*/Fine Powder fruit *of* *'Awla'*	Oral Intake Locally apply on hair/scalp

Dandruff

1	2	3	4	5
1.	Mustard oil + Curd		Mustard oil is mixed with curd	Locally apply on hair/scalp

Hair Fall and Regrowth

1	2	3	4	5
1.		Dodder (*'Gaas-Bel'*)	Mashed fruit of Dodder (*'Gaas-Bel'*)	Locally apply on scalp

ACUTE CONDITIONS

Fever

Sl. No.	*Home remedy Used*		*Method of Preparation*	
	Kitchen Medicine	*Medicinal Plant*	*Method of Preparation*	*Method of Use*
1	2	3	4	5
1.	Ginger+cardamom + Black Pepper + Carom Seeds (*'Ajwayan'*) + Fenugreek (*'Methi'*) + old jaggery		Boiled in water to make decoction	Oral Intake
2.		Eucalyptus (*'Sapheda'*)	Leaves of Eucalyptus (*'Sapheda'*) boiled in water for Vapourization	Vapour Inhalation
3.	Cloth		Cloth dipped in cold water	Cloth kept on the head and forehead
4.		Leaves of *'Tulsi'* + Smooth Angelica	Leaves of *'Tulsi'* + Smooth Angelica (*'Chora'*) + Chirette	Oral Intake

1	2	3	4	5
		(*'Chora'*) + Chirette Plant (*'Chiraita'*)	Plant (*'Chiraita'*) boiled in water to make decoction	
5.	Cumin Seeds (*'Jeera'*) +Rock (*'Gumma'*) salt + Cardamom	Young leaves of Tamarisk (*'Jhau'*) + leaves of Five Leaved Chaste (*'Vana'*) + Sweet Flag Root (*'Varaya'*)	All these ingredients are mixed together to make tablets	Oral Intake
6.	Turmeric	Rose + leaves of Holy Basil (*'Tulsi'*) + Margosa (*'Neem'*) Leaves	Turmeric with all plants in medicinal plant column boiled in 5 glasses of water to make it half of original quantity to make decoction	Oral Intake
7.	Cardamom + black pepper + Rock (*'Gumma'*) Salt	Holy Basil (*'Tulsi'*) *leaves* + Fennel Seeds (*'Saunph)'* + Sweet Violet (*'Vanaksha'*)	Ingredients in kitchen medicine column and plants mentioned in medicinal plant column boiled in water to make decoction	Oral Intake

1	2	3	4	5
8.	Cardamom + Black Pepper, + Ginger + Rock (*'Gumma'*) Salt + Dry Ginger (*'Sund'*) + Fenugreek (*'Methi'*) + Fennel Seeds (*'Saunph'*)	Holy Basil (*'Tulsi') leaves* + Sweet Violet (*'Vanaksha'*)	Ingredients in kitchen medicine column and plants mentioned in medicinal plant column boiled in water to make decoction	Oral Intake

Fever with Chills and Rigors: Malaria

Sl. No.	*Home remedy Used*		*Method of Preparation*	
	Kitchen Medicine	*Medicinal Plant*	*Method of Preparation*	*Method of Use*
1.		*'Pedara'*	Leaves of *'Pedera'* boiled in water to make decoction	Oral Consumption

Backache

Sl. No.	Home remedy Used		Method of Preparation	
	Kitchen Medicine	Medicinal Plant	Method of Preparation	Method of Use
1	2	3	4	5
1.		*'Kaila'* + *'Sankheru'*	Oil of *'Kaila'* and *'Sankheru'*	Massage to affected area
2.	Dry Ginger *('Sund')*		Dry Ginger *('Sund')* is roasted in clarified butter or *'Ghee'* and taken with milk	Oral Intake
3.		*'Sankheran'*	oil of *'Sankheran'*	Massage to affected area

Headache

Sl. No.	Kitchen Medicine	Medicinal Plant	Method of Preparation	Method of Use
1.	Fenugreek *('Methi')* + Fennel Seeds *('Saunph')* + Carom Seeds *('Ajwayan')*		A boiled in water to make decoction	Oral Intake
2.	Carom Seeds *('Ajwayan')* + Ginger + Big and Small Cardamom		A boiled in water to make decoction	Oral Intake

1	2	3	4	5
3.	Dry Ginger *('Sundi')* + Curd		Curd is used to make *'Lassi'* and scrubbed *'Sundi'* is added to make paste	Paste applied to affected area
4.	Dried coriander seeds *('Dhanyak')*	*'Beehan'*	Kitchen Medicine + Medicinal Plant roasted and crushed to make a paste with water.	Paste applied to affected area
5.	Mustard oil	Malbar Nut tree *('Basuti')* leaves	Hot mustard oil is applied on *'Basuti'* leaves	Tied around the head
6.	Dry Ginger *('Sundi')* + Mustard	Arungula *('Taramira')*	crushed together and mixed in *'Lassi'* made of curd	Paste applied to affected area

Bodyache

1.	Nutmeg *('Jaiphal')* + *'Ghee'*		Nutmeg *('Jaiphal')* is roasted in clarified butter *('Ghee')*	Oral Intake with Milk
2.	Dry Ginger *('Sund')* + *'Sinchar* salt' + Rock *('Gumma')* Salt + Black Pepper		Ingredients are mixed together in water	Oral Intake

1	2	3	4	5
3.	*Fennel Seeds ('Saunph')* + Fenugreek *('Methi')*		A + B boiled together in water to make decoction	Oral Intake
4.		*'Sankheru'*	Oil of *'Sankheru'*	Massage of the affected area

Stomach ache

1	2	3	4	5
1.	Fenugreek *('Methi')* seeds			Oral Intake with water
2.	Fennel Seeds *('Saunph')*			Oral Intake with water
3.	*Horse Gram ('Kullath dal')* Pulse			Oral Intake
4.		Mint leaves	Mint leaves are crushed and made into tablets	Oral Intake with water
5.	Almonds			Oral Intake with water
6.		*'Dhaansoa'*		Oral Intake
7.	Carom Seeds *('Ajwain')* + Peppermint		The extract of Carom Seeds *('Ajwain')* and Peppermint is mixed with a drop of water	Oral Intake
8.		Indian Gooseberry *('Awla')* + Belliric Myrobalan	Powder of Indian Gooseberry *('Awla')* + Belliric Myrobalan *('Baheda')* + Chebulei *('Harad')*	Oral Intake with warm water

1	2	3	4	5
		('Baheda') + Chebulei *('Harad')*		
9.	Asafetida		Powder of Asafetida	Oral Intake with warm water
10.	Turmeric Powder		Powder of Turmeric	Oral Intake with warm water
11.	Carom Seeds *('Ajwain')* + Fenugreek Seeds *('Methi')* + Fennel Seeds *('Saunph')*		A boiled together in water to make decoction	Oral Intake
12.	Cloves		Cloves are roasted	Oral Intake with cold water

Injuries

1	2	3	4	5
1.	Onion covering + Rock Salt *('Gumma namak')*		A paste is made by mixing crushed onion coverings and *'Gumma salt'*	Paste applied to affected area
2.	Milk	*'Shilajeet'*	*'Shilajeet'* is mixed in milk	Oral Intake
3.	Milk + Turmeric Powder		Turmeric Powder is added to hot milk	Oral Intake

Wound

1	2	3	4	5
1.		*'Durgadi'*	Leaves of *'Durgadi'* crushed to make paste	Paste applied to affected area
2.	Turmeric Powder + Mustard oil		Turmeric mixed in mustard oil	Local application on wound
3.	Turmeric Powder		Powder of Turmeric	Applied on the wounds

Cuts

1	2	3	4	5
1.	Cloth		Cloth piece is burnt to form ash	Ash filled in the cut
2.	Kerosene oil + Alum (*'Phitkari'*)			Kerosene oil or *'Phitkari'* applied on the cut

Burns

Sl. No.	*Home remedy Used*		*Method of Preparation*		*Specific Benefit*
	Kitchen Medicine	*Medicinal Plant*	*Method of Preparation*	*Method of Use*	
1.		Potato	Raw potato scrubbed to make paste	Paste is applied over the burnt	Relief from the burning sensation and to prevent formation of boils.
2.	Mustard oil	Mountain Eboy (*'Karal'*)	The bark of Mountain Eboy (*'Karal'*) is crushed and mixed with mustard oil to make a paste.	Paste is applied over the burnt	Provides relief. It promotes the healing process and also prevents scar formation.
3.	Cucumber (*'Kakadi'*)		The juice of Cucumber	Applied over the burnt area	Prevent burning sensation and formation of boils.
4.	Coconut oil			Coconut oil is applied over the burnt area	Prevent burning sensation and formation of boils
5.	Honey			Honey is applied over the burnt area	Heals the burns and prevents scar formation too.

Poisoning or Badalvish

Sl. No.	*Home remedy Used*		*Method of Preparation*	
	Kitchen Medicine	*Medicinal Plant*	*Method of Preparation*	*Method of Use*
1.	Ginger + Garlic + Black Pepper + Fenugreek Seeds *('Methi')*		Crushed together	Oral Intake
2.		*'Bukar'*	The leaves of *'Bukar'* are crushed to extract juice and mixed with water	Oral Intake
3.	Black Pepper		Powder of Black pepper	Oral Intake with cold water
4.	Fuller's earth		Fuller's earth mixed with cold water	Locally applied to affected area
5.		*'Bukar'*	*'Bukar'* is cooked and made into a vegetable dish	Oral Intake

Indigestion of Milk in Children

Sl. No.	*Home remedy Used*		*Method of Preparation*	
	Kitchen Medicine	*Medicinal Plant*	*Method of Preparation*	*Method of Use*
1.	Cardamom + Sugar + Carom Seeds (*'Ajwain'*)	Sweet Violet (*'Vanaksha'*)	Carom Seeds (*'Ajwain'*) is soaked in water and roasted on drying then mixed with Sweet Violet (*'Vanaksha'*) and Cardamom. This mixture is mixed in oiled water. Sugar is added	Oral Intake

Annexure 2(b)

Medicinal Plant Names—Himachal Pradesh

Vernacular Name	*English Name*	*Sanskrit Name*	*Botanical Name*
Aadu	Peach	*Amritam*	*Prunus persica*
Aliya	Garcinia	*Amlavetas*	*Garcinia pedunculata*
Chiraita	Chirette Plant	*Kirattikta*	*Andrographis paniculata*
Chitra	Lead Wart	*Chitrak*	*Plumbago zeylanica*
Chora	Smooth Angelica	*Chorak*	*Angelica glauca*
Chuara	Dry Date	*Pind Khajur*	*Phenix dactylifefra*
Gaas Bel	Dodder	*Amarvel*	*Cuscuta reflexa*
Gandhela	Curry leaf	*Girinimba/Krishnaninmba*	*Murraya koeniggi*

Vernacular Name	*English Name*	*Sanskrit Name*	*Botanical Name*
Jhau	Tamarisk	*Shavak*	*Tamarrix gallica*
Jufa	Hyssop	*Jupha*	*Hyssopus officinalis*
Kakad singi	Wax Tree/Japanese Tallow	*Karkatsringi*	*Rhus succedania*
Kamarkas	Flame of Forest	*Palash*	*Salvia plebeian*
Karal	Mountain Eboy	*Chanchanar*	*Bauhinia variegata*
Karela	Bitter Gourd	*Karvellak*	*Momordica*
Kasmale	Indian berberry	*Daruharidra*	*Berberis aristata*
Kharbuja	Musk Melon	*Amrutam*	*Cucumis melo*
Mulabi	Licorice	*Yashtimadhu*	*Glycyrrhiza glabra*
Pangaru	Indian Coral Tree	*Paribhadra*	*Erythrina variegata*
Suran	Telgu Potato, Elephant's Foot	*Suran/Arshoghna*	*Amorphophallus campanulatus*
Taramira	Arungula	*Bhutang*	*Eruca sativa*
Tali	Sheesham	*Agru*	*Dalbergia sissoo*
Vanaksha	Wild/Sweet Violet	*Vanaspika*	*Viola odorata*
Varaya	Sweet Flag Root	*Vacha*	*Acorus calamus*
Vasuti	Malbar Nut	*Vasa*	*Adathoda vesica*

Annexure 3(a)

Home Remedies, Sagar District—Madhya Pradesh

Name of the Ailment	*Type of Home Remedy*	*Method of Preparation and Usage*
1	2	3
Cough		
1.	Ginger + Holy Basil (*'Tulsi'*)	5 grams of Ginger with 4-5 leaves of *'Tulsi'* is mixed with tea and taken 4-5 times in a day.
2.	Sanjivani Tablet *('Sanjivani Vati')* + Honey	Sanjivani Tablet *('Sanjivani Vati')* (Ayurvedic medicine) (1 spoon) mixed with honey and taken.
3.	Roasted Ginger + Clove (*'Lavang')*+ Honey/Sugar	5-6 grams roasted Ginger and Cloves (*'Lavang')* are mixed with sugar or Honey and taken.
4.	Ginger + Garlic fried + Clarified	2-4 cloves of Garlic along with Ginger is crushed and fried

1	2	3
	Butter *('Ghee')*	in 2-3 spoons of clarified butter (*Ghee*) and taken.
5.	Peacock feather + Honey	Peacock feather is burnt and mixed with honey and taken.
6.	Turmeric powder + Jaggery	1-2 spoons of Turmeric powder is roasted and mixed with Jaggery and taken before going to bed in the night. Drinking water after that night is prohibited.
7.	Extract from bark of *Babul* *('Babool')* + Extract from bark of Sponge Tree *('Kandi')* tree + Milk + Water	Extracts from the bark of *Babul* *('Babool')* and Sponge Tree *('Kandi')* tree is put in water and crushed to get the extracts. Half a cup of this extract is mixed with half a glass of milk and taken.
8.	Ripe fruit of *'Bokbillaiya'* + Seeds of Marking Nut *('Bhilma')* + Honey + Sugar	The ripe fruit of *'Bokbillaiya'* and the seeds of Marking Nut *('Bhilma')* are roasted in fire and crushed. It is then mixed with sugar or honey and taken. Dosage is 1-2 spoons, twice a day
9.	Mango leaves	A spoonful of Warm extract of Mango leaves is taken.
10.	Betel leaves	Betel leaves are chewed
11.	*'Lakhera's 'Mahi'* + Honey	*'Lakhera's 'Mahi'* is burnt and mixed with a spoonful of honey and taken.
12.	Pomegranate fruit	The outer covering of Pomegranate fruit is chewed.
13.	Roasted Ginger + Jaggery	5 grams of roasted Ginger is mixed with 5-10 grams of jaggery and taken.

1	2	3
Cold		
1.	Holy Basil Leaves (*'Tulsi'*) leaves + Ginger	Tea made with Holy Basil Leaves (*'Tulsi'*) leaves and Ginger is taken.
2.	Roasted Ginger + Garlic + Jaggery	2-4 cloves of Garlic and 5-10 grams of Ginger are roasted and mixed with 5-10 grams of jaggery and taken.
3.	Turmeric + Jaggery + Boiled Milk	One spoon Turmeric powder and jaggery is boiled with one glass of milk and taken before going to bed.
4.	*'Karench'* + Honey	1-2 seeds of the fruit of *'Karench'* are roasted and taken with honey. Dosage is twice for 2-3 days. It can be taken without honey too.
5.	Roasted Asafetida + Roasted Dry Ginger (*'Saunth'*)	Roasted Asafetida with roasted Dry Ginger (*'Saunth'*) is crushed and taken with honey or sugar. Syrup is taken for 2-3 days.
6.	Roots of Castor Oil plant (*'Andi'*) +Milk + Water	The juice extracted from crushed Castor Oil plant (*'Andi'*) roots is mixed with one cup milk or half a glass of water and taken.
7.	Urine of Cow (*'Gau-Mutra'*)	Children below the age of one are given a spoonful of Cow's urine (*'Gou-Mutra'*), 2-3 days in a week to prevent catching cold.
8.	Roasted Black Pepper + Clove +	Roasted Black Pepper and Clove is crushed and taken with

1	2	3
	Sugar Syrup	sugar syrup.
9.	Cloves + Pepper (*'Lendi Pipali'*) + Honey	Roasted cloves and Pepper *('Lendi Peeper')* is crushed and taken with honey.
10.	*Babul* (*'Babool')* tree + Honey + Water	The bark and flowers of *Babul* (*'Babool')* tree are mixed with water, crushed and sieved using cloth. 2-3 spoonful of this extract is mixed with honey and taken twice daily.
11.	The viscous liquid from the Silk Worm + Honey	1-2 drops viscous liquid of the insides of Silk-Worm is mixed with 2-4 drops honey and given twice a day to small children.
Fever		
1.	Leaves of Lemon *('Nimbuk')* + Margosa (*'Neem')* + Tinospora (*'Gurbel')* + Water	Lemon leaves, Margosa (*'Neem')* leaves and Tinospora (*'Gurbel')* are boiled in a glass of water. When it is reduced to a cup of decoction, the decoction is taken twice daily for 3-4 days. It is good for malarial fever as well as other types of fevers.
2.	Castor Oil Plant (*'Andi')* tree + Water	The leaves of Castor Oil Plant (*'Andi')* tree are crushed and the extract is mixed with water and taken.
3.	The extract from the roots of *'Idulan'* + Sugar	The root of *'Idulan'* is boiled and a cup of the concoction with sugar is taken daily for 2-3 days.

1	2	3
4.	Margosa (*'Neem'*) leaves + Sugar	Margosa (*'Neem'*) leaves from two twigs boiled to make decoction and sugar is added and taken for 3 days.
Dysentery		
1.	Jambol (*'Jamun'*) + Water + Sugar	The outer covering of bark of Jamun (*'Jamun'*) tree crushed with water to make juice. Sugar added in this juice. This juice is taken in quantity of ½-1 glass.
2.	*Bael* (*'Bel'*) + Cumin Seeds + Sugar	Drink made of pulp of Bael (*'Bel'*), Cumin Seeds (*'Jeera'*) and Sugar is beneficial.
3.	Indian Gooseberry (*'Anwla'*) + Sugar	The outer covering of Indian Gooseberry (*'Anwla'*) tree is crushed and the juice is mixed with sugar and taken.
4.	Indian Flame Tree (*'Palash'*) + Milk + Sugar	The outer covering of Indian Flame Tree (*'Palash'*) fruit is crushed and the juice extracted is mixed with milk and sugar and taken.
5.	Arjuna (*'Koha'*) + Sandal Chariot (*'Tinsa'*) + Milk + Sugar	The outer covering of Arjuna (*'Koha'*) and Sandal Chariot (*'Tinsa'*) fruits are crushed and the juice extracted is mixed with milk and sugar or date-sugar and taken.
6.	Rice + Curd or Chapati + Buttermilk	-Rice with curd is taken for 1-2 days to cure dysentery. -Buttermilk with salt is taken or it is mixed with *Chappati* and taken.

1	2	3
7.	Tamarind leaves + Water	Fistful of crushed tamarind leaves are crushed with water to make extract and taken for 2-3 days.
8.	Mint leaves + Sugar/Date Sugar	Juice from 6-8 mint leaves are mixed with sugar or date-sugar and taken. Both whole leaves or juice of the leaves can be taken.
9.	Roasted Dry Ginger (*'Saunth'*) + Honey	Roasted and powdered Dry Ginger (*'Saunth'*) is mixed with 3-4 drops of honey and taken.
10.	Mango tree + Silk Cotton Tree (*'Semar'*) + Date Sugar + Water	The juice extracted from the outer covering of bark of Mango or fruit of Silk Cotton Tree (*'Semar'*) is mixed with water and date-sugar and taken.
11.	Roots of *'Suleha'* or *'Vyakul'* + Milk	Roots of *'Suleha'* and *'Vyakul'* are crushed and the juice extracted is mixed with a cup of milk and date-sugar and taken for 10-15 days.
12.	Box Myrtle (*'Aar'*)	Crushed root of Box Myrtle (*'Aar'*) is taken.

1	2	3
Vomiting and Nausea		
1.	Burnt big Cardamom + Honey	Big Cardamom is burnt and a fine powder of the crushed Cardamom is mixed with a spoonful of honey and taken at an interval of 1-2 hours throughout the day.
2.	Mint leaves + Sugar.	Mint leaves are crushed and taken with sugar.
3.	*'Mahi of Lakhera'*	*'Mahi of Lakhera'* is mixed in water and taken.
		'Mahi of Lakhera' is burnt and mixed with 2-3 drops of honey and taken twice or thrice in a day.
4.	Stem of Peacock + Honey	Stem of Peacock-feather is burnt and mixed with spoonful of honey and taken 2-4 times in a day.
5.	Cumin seeds (*'Jeera'*) + Black salt	Crushed seeds of Cumin (*'Jeera'*) is taken with black salt
6.	Betel nut *('Supari')*	Betel nut *('Supari')* is sucked on.
7.	ORS mixture + Water.	A glass of water with 2-3 spoonfuls of sugar and a pinch of salt is taken. ORS mixture provided by the AWW or ASHA is taken.
8.	Juice of Onion + Sugar	A spoonful of onion juice is mixed with sugar and taken.
9.	Jambol seeds (*'Jamun')* + Honey	1-2 burnt seeds of seeds of Jambol (*'Jamun')* are mixed with 2-4 drops of honey and taken.
10.	Ginger + Honey	Juice of Ginger is mixed with honey and taken.

1	2	3
Headache		
1.	Leaves of Eucalyptus	Leaves of Eucalyptus are crushed and applied.
2.	Aloe Vera (*'Gavar Patha'*)	Pulp *('Bakla')* of Aloe Vera (*'Gavar Patha')* is tied.
3.	Piece of cloth.	The head is tied tightly with a piece of cloth or towel.
4.	Mustard seeds + Cloves + Water	Mustard seeds and Cloves are crushed and mixed with water. This paste is applied on the head.
5.	Ginger	Ginger tea is taken.
6.	Sandalwood + Cold Water	A stick of Sandalwood is scrubbed on a piece of stone and a paste is made by mixing Sandalwood with cold water and applied on the head.
7.	Rice Plant leaves *('Vihi')* + Basil leaves *('Tulsi')* + Asthma Plant (*'Doodhghass')* grass	Rice Plant leaves *('Vihi'),* Basil leaves *('Tulsi')* and Asthma Plant (*'Doodhghass')* grass crushed together and paste is applied on head.
8.	Black soil + Water	Paste of Black soil and water is applied.
9.	Ginger	Drops of Ginger juice is put inside the nostrils.
10.	Leaves of Peepal or Sacred Fig *('Pipal')* + Water	Leaves of Peepal or Sacred Fig *('Pipal')* tree are crushed and a paste is made with water. This paste is applied on the head.
11.	Leaves of *'Ashpake'* + Water	Leaves of *'Ashpake'* are crushed and mixed with water. This paste is applied on the head.
12.	Leaves of Guava (*'Amrud'*)	Leaves of Guava (*'Amrud'*) are crushed and applied on the head.

1	2	3
Bodyache		
1.	Mustard oil + Garlic + Fenugreek (*'Methi'*)	50 grams mustard oil is mixed with 3-4 cloves of Garlic and 10 grams Fenugreek (*'Methi'*) seeds. This oil is warmed and used for massaging.
2.	Kerosene oil	Massage using Kerosene oil is done.
3.	Warm Brick or hot water + Salt	Bathing or fomentation is done using warm brick or hot water mixed with salt.
4.	*Andagua'*leaves + 'Clarified Butter	Fomentation is done with clarified butter applied using warm *'Andagua'* leaves.
5.	*'Karkichyai'*	Wet roots of *'Karkichyai'* is scrubbed, dried and applied.
6.	*'Baganthu'*	*'Baganthu'* is mixed with warm mustard oil and applied on the affected area.
7.	Seeds of Thorn Apple plant (*'Dhatura'*) + Mustard oil	Seeds of Thorn Apple plant (*'Dhatura'*) are heated in mustard oil and applied.
8.	Asafoetida (*'Hing'*)	Asafoetida (*'Hing'*) is heated in water and applied.

1	2	3
Backache		
1.	Garlic + Fenugreek (*'Methi'*) + Mustard oil	50 grams mustard oil is mixed with 3-4 cloves of garlic and 10 grams Fenugreek (*'Methi'*) seeds. This oil is heated and used for massaging.
2.	Asafoetida (*'Hing'*) + Water	Asafoetida (*'Hing'*) is heated in water and applied.
3.	Kerosene oil	Massage with kerosene oil is done.
4.	Brick or Warm Water	Fomentation using warm brick or warm water is done.
5.	Thorn Apple (*'Dhatura'*) seeds + Mustard Oil	Thorn Apple (*'Dhatura'*) seeds are mixed and heated in Mustard oil and applied.
6.	Leaves of Pull Back (*'Ankua'*) or Aconite (*'Bariya'*) + Urine of Sheep	Leaves of Pull Back (*'Ankua'*) or Aconite (*'Bariya'*) are mixed in the urine of sheep and fomentation is done using this liquid, applied by the means of leaves.
7.	Wet roots of *'Karkichyai'*	Wet roots of *'Karkichyai'* are scrubbed, dried and applied.

1	2	3
Joint Pain		
1.	*'Baganthu'* + Mustard oil	Pieces of *'Baganthu'* are boiled in Mustard oil and the oil is applied on the affected area.
2.	Roasted Asafoetida (*'Gathua'* or *Hing)* + Fragrant Screw Pine (*'Kev')* + Jaggery	Roasted Asafoetida (*'Gathua'* or *Hing)* and Screw Pine (*'Kev')* are roasted in fire, mixed in jaggery and taken in the morning and evening daily to cure joint pain.
3.	Castor Seed (*'Andi'* or *'Aerand')* oil	Fomentation is done with warm Ricinus Seed (*'Andi'* or *'Aerand')* oil, applied using leaves over the affected area.
4.	Juice of leaves of Drum Stick (*'Munga')* plant	Snacks mixed with the juice of Drum Stick (*'Munga')* plant leaves are taken.
5.	Old lime (calcium carbonate)	Old lime (calcium carbonate) is applied over the affected area.
6.	Thorn Apple *('Dhatura')* seeds + Mustard oil	Thorn Apple *('Dhatura')* seeds are mixed and heated in mustard oil and applied.
7.	*'Thoobar'* having *'Kos'* + Mustard oil	*'Thoobar'* having *'Kos'* is boiled in Mustard oil and this oil is applied over the affected area.
8.	Box Myrtle (*'Kaiphal'*) + Mustard	Fine powder outer covering of bark of Box Myrtle (*'Kaiphal'*) is mixed in warm Mustard oil is used for massage and for local application.
9.	Asafoetida (*'Gathua')* + Water	Water in which Asafoetida (*'Gathua')* is added is used for bathing.

1	2	3
Constipation		
1.	Carom Seeds (*'Ajwain'*) + Salt	Carom Seeds (*'Ajwain'*) mixed with salt is taken.
2.	Guava (*'Amrud'*)	Boiled Guava (*'Amrud'*) is eaten.
3.	Buttermilk + Salt or Black salt	Buttermilk mixed with salt or Black salt is taken.
4.	Crushed Carom Seeds (*'Ajwain'*) + Fenugreek seeds (*'Methi'*) + Jaggery	Crushed Carom Seeds (*'Ajwain'*) and Fenugreek seeds (*'Methi'*) seeds are roasted, mixed with jaggery and taken.
5.	Dried Chebulei (*'Harad'*) + Castor (*'Andi'*) oil	Dried Chebulei (*'Harad'*) 2-4 dried roasted in Castor (*'Andi'*) oil or mixed with black salt is eaten at night.
6.	Leaves of Jambol (*'Jamun'*)	Leaves of Jambol (*'Jamun'*) are eaten.
7.	Lemon (*'Nimbu'*) + Black Salt	Lemon slices mixed with Black Pepper and Black Salt are kept overnight and taken on an empty stomach the next morning.
8.	Baking Soda	Half a spoon of Baking Soda mixed with water is taken.
9.	*'Triphala Churna'* (*'Harad + Behda+ Awala'*) (Ayurvedic preparation)	A spoonful of *'Triphala Churna'* is mixed with a glass of warm water and taken at night before going to bed.

1	2	3
Stomachache		
1.	Coram Seeds *('Ajwain')*	Coram Seeds *('Ajwain')* is taken.
2.	Mustard oil	Stomach is massaged using Mustard oil.
3.	Black Thorn Apple *('Dhatura')*	Black Thorn Apple *('Dhatura')* is taken.
4.	Root of *'Rundulan'* or seed of Desert Date *('Igua')* + Jaggery	Root of *'Rundulan'* or seed of Desert Date *('Igua')* is mixed in jaggery and taken.
5.	Fenugreek *('Methi')* seeds	Boiled Fenugreek *('Methi')* seeds are added to vegetables and consumed.
6.	Root of *'Kattara'* + Jaggery	Root of *'Kattara'* is mixed with jaggery and taken.
7.	Pill made of lime (calcium carbonate) + Jaggery	Pill made of lime (calcium carbonate) mixed with jaggery is taken.
8.	Leaves of Jambol *('Jamun')* or Rice plant *('Vihi')* + Carom Seeds *('Ajwain')* + Black Salt	Leaves of Jambol *('Jamun')* or Rice plant *('Vihi')* are mixed with Carom Seeds *('Ajwain')* and black salt and crushed together. This mixture is eaten to cure stomachache.
Itching		
1.	Margosa *('Neem')* leaves + Water	Margosa *('Neem')* leaves are added in water and this water is used for bathing.
2.	Cow dung + Cow's urine	Hands are washed using Cow dung and Cow's urine in the

1	2	3
		cattle-shed.
3.	Sulphur (*'Gandhak'*) + *'Hariya Thutha'* + Oil of *Mitti*	Sulphur (*'Gandhak'*) and *'Hariya Thuta'* are boiled in Oil of *Mitti* and applied.
4.	Burnt bee-hive + Oil	Burnt bee-hive is mixed with oil and applied.
5.	Seeds of Thorn Apple (*'Dhatura'*)	Seeds of Thorn Apple (*'Dhatura'*) are crushed and applied.

Skin Problems

1.	Holy Basil (*'Tulsi'*) leaves + Bark of Margosa (*'Neem'*) tree + Water	2-3 Holy Basil (*'Tulsi'*) leaves mixed with water and bark of Margosa (*'Neem'*) tree are crushed together and applied.
2.	Cow dung + Cow's urine	Cow dung mixed with cow's urine is applied.
3.	Leaves of Opium (*'Afu'*) plant + Water	Leaves of Opium (*'Aphu'*) plant are boiled in water and this water is used for bathing
4.	Chiraunji Nut Tree (*'Chiraul'*) extract	3-4 leaves of *Chiraunji* Nut Tree (*'Chiraul'*) are crushed and the extract is applied over the affected area.
5.	Leaves of Trailing Eclipta (*'Ghamra'*)	Leaves of Trailing Eclipta (*'Ghamra'*) are crushed and applied.
6.	Leaves of Lablab Bean (*'Sem'*)	Leaves of Lablab Bean (*'Sem'*) are crushed and applied.
7.	Coconut oil + Camphor	Coconut oil mixed with camphor is applied.

1	2	3
Tonic for Strength		
1.	Clarified butter (*Ghee*) + Milk	Clarified butter (*Ghee*) added in milk is taken.
2.	Unripe *'Deval'* + Honey + Milk + Water	Unripe *'Deval'* kept overnight in water is mixed with milk and honey and taken.
3.	*'Gulakhiri'*	*'Gulakhiri'* is crushed and taken.
4.	Winter Cherry (*'Bach Ashwagandha'*)	Selected Winter Cherry (*'Bach Ashwagandha'*) is crushed and taken.
5.	Roots of Trailing Eclipta (*'Ganerua'*) + *'Chue'*	Roots of Trailing Eclipta (*'Ganerua'*) and *'Chue'* are crushed together and taken.
6.	Roots of *'Ughaar'* + Milk	Roots of *'Ughaar'* are crushed and mixed with milk and taken.
7.	*'Shankargheri'* + Milk	Paste of *'Shankargheri'* is mixed with milk and taken.
8.	*'Saunth'* +Asparagus (*'Satavar'*) + Black Pepper + Clarified Butter (*Ghee*) + Milk + Honey.	A mixture of *'Saunth'*, Asparagus (*'Satavar'*) and Black Pepper mixed in clarified butter (*Ghee*) is taken with milk and honey.
9.	Seeds of *'Madarmach'* + Flower (*'Dubri'*) of Butter Tree (*'Mahua'*)	50-60 gram seeds of *'Madarmach'* is mixed with Flower (*'Dubri'*) of Butter Tree (*'Mahua'*) and taken for gaining strength.
10.	Sprouted Bengal gram (*'Bangali Chane'*) + Jaggery	Sprouted Bengal (*'Bangali Chane'*) gram jaggery and taken.
11.	Crushed White Gourd (*'Saphed*	Crushed white gourd (*'Saphed Dudha'*) mixed with milk is

1	2	3
	Dudha') + Milk	taken.
12.	Winter cherry (*'Asagandh')* + Sprouted wheat	Mixture made of crushed Winter cherry (*'Aswagandha')* mixed with sprouted wheat is taken.
Gynaecological Problems		
1.	Roots of *'Ughaar'* + Water	Crushed roots of *'Ughaar'* is mixed with water and taken.
2.	Leaves of Chiraungi Nut Tree (*'Chirauji')* + Water	Crushed leaves of Chiraungi Nut Tree (*'Chirauji')* are mixed with water and taken.
3.	*'Maghvari'* + Sugar	*'Maghvari'* is cut and dried. Its fine powder is mixed with sugar and taken.
4.	Crushed *'Karai Chench'* + Milk	Crushed *'Karai Chench'* is mixed with milk and taken.
5.	Seeds of *'Madramachch'*+ Flower (*'Dabri')* of Butter Tree (*'Mahua')* + *'Vada Magerua'*+ fine powder of the wood of *'Meghi'* + Asparagus (*'Satavar')*	A mixture of the seeds of *'Madramachch'*, Flower (*'Dabri')* of Butter Tree (*'Mahua')*, *'Vada Magerua'*, fine powder of the wood of *'Meghi'* and Asparagus (*'Satavar')* is made. This mixture is either added to rice pudding or a spoonful of this mixture is taken twice daily with a glass of milk and Palm-sugar.
6.	Flowers of Hibiscus (*'Jaasoun'*) + Roots of Thatch Grass Plant	1-2 crushed flowers of Hibiscus (*'Jaasoun'*), crushed roots of Thatch Grass Plant (*'Kaans')* in water are mixed with milk

1	2	3
	(*'Kaans'*) + Water + Milk	and taken
7.	Jaggery + Fenugreek (*'Methi'*) + Carom Seeds (*'Ajwain'*) + Dry Ginger (*'Saunth'*)	Jaggery, Fenugreek (*'Methi'*), Carom Seeds (*'Ajwain'*) and Dry Ginger (*'Saunth'*) are roasted and mixed together to make *'Laddoos'*.
8.	Leaves of Henna (*'Mehndi'*) plant + Honey	For abortion 8-10 leaves of Henna (*'Mehndi'*) plant are crushed and mixed with honey and taken till the foetus is aborted.
9.	Warm water	Massage of the abdominal region is done using warm water, to relieve pain.
10.		Proper cleanliness and hygiene of the private parts is maintained.
Cuts and Wounds		
1.	The bark of Bael (*'Bilja'*) + Water	The bark of Bael (*'Bilja'*) is crushed with water. This paste is applied over the wound.
2.	Black Catechu (*'Kattha'*)	Black Catechu (*'Kattha'*) is applied over the wound for 3-5 days.
3.	The bark of Indian Liquorice (*'Gunja'*)	The bark of Indian Liquorice (*'Gunja'*) is crushed and applied over the wound and a piece of cloth is tied over it.
4.	The extract of Trailing Eclipta	The extract of Trailing Eclipta (*'Ghamra'*) is applied over the

1	2	3
	('Ghamra')	wound.
5.	Turmeric powder +clarified butter (*Ghee*)	Turmeric powder mixed with clarified butter (*Ghee*) is applied over the wound.
6.	Alum *('Geru')*	Alum *('Geru')* or Alum is applied over the wound.
7.	Onion pieces + Clarified butter (*Ghee*)	Onion pieces fried in clarified butter (*Ghee*) are tied over the wound with a piece of cloth.
8.	Spreading Hogweed *('Patharcha')*	Spreading Hogweed *('Patharcha')* is crushed and applied over the wound.
9.	*'Langhan'* + Oil	*'Langhan'* mixed with oil is applied.
Unconsciousness		
1.	Socks	The patient is made to smell socks.
2.		The chest is massaged.
3.	Onion juice	Onion juice is put into the nostrils.
4.		Certain magico-religious rituals are followed to bring the patient back to consciousness.
5.	Black Pepper powder	Small quantity of Black Pepper powder is put into the nostrils.
6.	Box myrtle/Bayberry *('Kaiphal')*	Box myrtle/Bayberry *('Kaiphal')* is rubbed over the body and small quantity of Bayberry *('Kaiphal')* is put into the nostrils.

1	2	3
7.	Cold Water.	The face is washed with cold water.
8.	*'Jatun'* flowers + Water or Milk	Crushed *'Jatun'* flowers are mixed with water or milk and taken.
Jaundice		
1.	Sugarcane juice	Sugarcane juice is taken. Certain magico-religious rituals are also followed for treating Jaundice.
2.	Leaves of *'Chuhar'* + *'Gaakar'*	The leaves of *'Chuhar'* are kept in *'Gaakar'*, warmed and eaten.
3.	*'Kaheera'* seeds + Milk	*'Kaheera'* seeds mixed in milk are taken.
4.	The seeds of Papaya + Copper coin	The seeds of Papaya are tied on the waist or stomach along with a copper coin.
5.	Radish (*'Muli'*)	Radish (*'Muli'*) is cooked and eaten.
6.	Aloe Vera *('Gwarpatha')*	*Aloe Vera ('Gwarpatha')* is taken.
7.	*'Daunth'* + Asparagus (*'Satavar'*) + Black Pepper + Sugar + Clarified butter (*Ghee*)	*'Daunth'*, Asparagus (*'Satavar'*), Black Pepper and sugar are mixed in clarified butter (*Ghee*) and taken daily in the morning.

1	2	3
Mental Stress and Prevention of Madness		
1.	Black *'Junar'* + Milk	To prevent madness after being bitten by a mad dog, black *'Junar'* mixed with milk is taken.
2.	Mint leaves + Lemon + Sugar	To relieve mental stress, water-based drink made of mint leaves, lemon, and sugar is taken. It is advised to take cooling food items to relieve stress.
3.	Bael *('Bel')*	Drinks made of the fruit of Bael *('Bel')* are taken.
Fractures		
1.	Veld Grape *('Hadjod')* + Goat's/ Cow's milk	Herb called as Veld Grape *('Hadjod')* is crushed and applied over the affected area. Goat's and cow's milk is taken to hasten the healing process.
2.	*'Chilo'*	Crushed *'Chilo'* is applied.

Ailment	*Home Remedies*
1. Menstrual problems	No home remedies available. Treatment at the hospital.
	Fomentation is done using hot brick wrapped in cloth.

Ailment	*Home Remedies*
	Crushed flowers of Hibiscus (*'Jasson'*) are mixed in milk or buttermilk and taken. Warm water, Carom Seeds (*'Ajwain'*), jaggery and Ginger tea are taken. Cleanliness and hygiene of the private parts is maintained
Diet and dietary restrictions during menstruation	
	Hot, spicy and sour food is avoided. Food that leads to gas formation is avoided. Lemon and sour food is also avoided.
Reason for problems	
	Weak stomach, weak liver and poor diet leads to menstrual problems. Some women have menstrual problems due to their natural body constitution or due to excessive body heat. Weakness and lack of blood.
2. Home remedies and traditional practices during pregnancy	Roasted and crushed Cumin Seeds (*'Jeera'*) is given to control vomiting. The *'Dais'* or experienced women give stomach massages using oil to cure stomachache during pregnancy. Hands and feet of the pregnant woman are massage by the *'Dais'*.
Diet and dietary restrictions and other restrictions during	All kinds of fruits and vegetables are taken. Strenuous work and lifting of heavy objects is prohibited.

Ailment	*Home Remedies*
pregnancy	
	During the 9th month of pregnancy social visits are reduced and the women do not cross rivers, streams etc.
	Food that leads to gas formation and hot spicy food is avoided.
	New clothes, accessories etc. are not used. Henna (*'Mehndi'*) is not applied.
Traditional practices and home remedies for safe and easy delivery	Husband's or nephew's right toe is washed and the water is drunk by the pregnant woman.
	Cow's urine is drunk by the pregnant woman.
	Curd is not eaten during pregnancy to avoid swelling in the body.
	Lord 'Mahaveer' is worshipped by the pregnant woman.
	Regular exercise by doing household work such as crushing of wheat and sweeping and swabbing the floor is done by the women to promote easy delivery.
	Cow dung is mixed with water and strained using a cloth piece and a spoonful of the extract is given to the pregnant woman.
	The holy waters of river Ganges and Narmada is stored with a copper coin immersed in it and this water is taken.
Diet	Oily, spicy, sour and gas-producing foods are avoided. Pulse especially *'Moong'*, milk, *'Dalia'*, *'Khedar Dalia'* and *'Khichadi'* are taken more.

Ailment	*Home Remedies*
Reasons for problem	Weakness of the body leads to difficult delivery.
Practices followed for a period of forty days after delivery	Bathing with boiling water in which Margosa (*'Neem'*) leaves have been added.
	Fomentation of the back with warm Margosa (*'Neem'*) leaves.
	Warm water is kept below *'Nitamb'*; and fomentation with warmed up leaves is done.
	Water of Tailed Pepper/Cubeb (*'Kanko'*) is taken.
	The head is kept tied.
	Carom Seeds (*'Ajwain'*) is burnt and fomentation is done with the smoke emanating from it.
	Massage with mustard oil is given.
	'Laddoos' made of *'Biswar'* and jaggery is taken.
	'Harira' is taken twice a day.
	'Dalia' and Sowa Millet (*'Sama'*) rice is taken.
	'Harira Ladoos' are taken for five days; milk and *'Dalia'* are taken for five days after that. Ten days after delivery *chapatti* with milk and *'Khichadi'* is taken.
	Spicy, oily, sour and gas-producing food is avoided. Light and easy to digest food is taken.

Ailment	*Home Remedies*
To maintain the good health of the new mother and to promote milk production	3-5 snails are crushed and mixed in milk on Sundays and Tuesdays and given to the new mother without informing her of the contents.
	Less *Chappati* and more *'Harira'* and jaggery are fed to the new mother.
	Green vegetables, Jaggery with *'Biswar'* and *'Dalia'* with milk is taken.
Reason for problem	Inadequate milk production in a new mother is linked to superstitious belief of punishment for the woman's sins.
Traditional practices of infant care	The infant is bathed with warm water and dried using a clean soft cloth immediately after birth.
	The infant is breast-fed by the mother, within half an hour to one hour after birth. If the mother does not produce milk, then cow's or goat's milk is given to the new born.
	The *'Dai'* or family members apply sweet oil to the New born's umbilical cord.
	Crushed *'Khapra'* is applied to the new born's umbilical cord.
	The new-born child is given massages twice daily for at least a month
	Wheat flour mixed with oil and Turmeric is kneaded and dough balls are made. These dough balls are used for massaging the new-born child for at least 2-3 days after birth, in order to remove dirt and impurities from

Ailment	Home Remedies
	the child's body.
Dietary restrictions for the lactating mother	Cold water, heavy food and gas-producing vegetables are to be avoided.
Traditional practices related to lactation and breast-feeding	The child is breast-fed while lying down in the mother's lap.
	During the evening the child is breast-fed while sitting in the mother's lap. The child is not laid down in the lap to avoid pain in the ears. The child is breast-fed up to one or one and a half to two years at least. If the woman gives birth to two children within two consecutive years then the milk produced is not enough for either of the children. If the mother does not lactate then the other lactating women of the family breast-feed the new-born, so that the child gets adequate nutrition.
Traditional practices related to introduction of solid food to the child	Once the child is 6-7 months old, the family members start giving small pieces of *Chappati*, milk, *'Dalia'* etc. to the child.
	Watery *'Sabudana'* and biscuits are also given. Solid food is given 3-4 times in a day to the child.

Ailment	*Home Remedies*
Introduction of drinking water to newborns	If the child is born in summers then water is given after the child is one month old and if the child is born in winters then water is given after 5-6 months.
	Some mothers start giving water to the new-born in 2-3 months itself.
Hygiene and promotion of good health related traditional practices followed for the new-born	Wheat flour mixed with oil and turmeric is kneaded and dough balls are made. These dough balls are used for massaging the new-born child, in order to remove dirt and impurities from the child's body. The child is given massage with mustard oil ad bathed with hot water. The child is bathed with Margosa (*'Neem'*) leaves boiled in water, 3-4 times a day for ten days after birth. Kohl is applied in the eyes of the child and the child is given massage with mustard oil.
Massage related practices	Massage is given to the child twice daily for two months after birth and then once daily till the child is a year old.
Child-care practices for the prevention and cure of illnesses	The children are clothed in warm clothes to protect them from cold. Crushed nutmeg is applied to the head and body of the children to prevent them from catching cold. Nutmeg keeps the body warm.

Ailment	*Home Remedies*
	Asafoetida paste and cow's urine is applied to prevent stomachache and cold.
	To protect the child from cold a mixture of roasted Turmeric, *'Juhaga'*, Box Myrtle *(Kaiphal)*, Musk *('Kasturi')* and Bamboo Manna *('Bansalochan')* is give along with mother's milk.
Symptoms that the child is not well	Excessive crying and declining feeds.
	Heavy breathing.
	Presses the area of pain.
Geriatric care	During illness medicines and light nutritious meal is given.
	Dietary care is taken.
	The old people at home are given massages daily.

Annexure 3(b)

Baiga Remedies, Sagar District—Madhya Pradesh

1.	**Ear-ache**: Extract of roasted Onion is put into the ear.
2.	**Pus formation in the ears**: Mustard oil is heated and drops of the oil are put into the ear.
3.	**Bad breath**: The outer covering of Pomegranate fruit is boiled in water and this water is used for gargling.
4.	**For strong teeth**: The flowers of Pomegranate are dried in the shade and crushed. This powder is used to clean the gums and teeth. It makes the teeth strong and prevents bleeding of the teeth and gums.
5.	**Burning sensation during urination**: • Crushed Onions are boiled in water. Once it has evaporated and concentrated to half the initial volume, then this extract is strained and cooled and given for at least two days. • Coriander seeds are crushed with water and taken for relief.
6.	**To cure stools with blood**: 10 gram Jambol (*'Jamun'*) seeds are crushed in water and the extract is sieved and taken twice daily.
7.	**Nocturnal emissions:** The covering of Pomegranate fruit is crushed and 5-10 grams is taken twice daily to prevent nocturnal emissions.
8.	**To cure excessive menstrual bleeding:** 10 gram bark of Jambol (*'Jamun'*) tree is boiled in 250 ml water. The extract is strained and taken twice daily to cure excessive menstrual bleeding.

9.	**Migraine:** The leaves of Carrot plant are boiled in water and the extract is put into the warm extract is put into the nose and ears drop-wise to cure migraine.
10.	**Cure from loo affliction:** • The leaves and fruits of raw Mango are boiled in water and mixed with sugar and taken to cure loo affliction. • Gram seeds and Henna (*'Mehndi'*) leaves are crushed together and applied on the body for relief.
11.	**On hurting the foot:** Fuller's earth *('Multani Mitti)* is applied on the toe nails and the hurt area to give relief.
12.	**Treatment of pimples:** 10 gram milk cream and Lemon juice is mixed and applied on the face. This improves the complexion and treats the pimples.
13.	**Tooth-ache:** • Lemon juice is mixed with crushed Cloves and the paste is applied on the teeth for relief from toothache. • Clove oil and Peppermint is applied over the affected area. • Alum is crushed and kept between the aching teeth. • Mustard oil mixed with salt is applied over the affected area. • Decoction made of Carom seeds (*'Ajwain')* and water is used for gargling.
14.	**Conjunctivitis:** • Marigold leaves are crushed and applied on the eyes. • Leaves of Rice Plant (*'Vihi')* is crushed and applied on the eyes. • Rose water or extract of rose petals or leaves or extract of the leaves of Lulab Bean (*'Sem'*) is put drop-wise into the eyes to cure conjunctivitis. • Drops of extract of Sickel Senna (*'Puar')* leaves and Honey are put into the eyes for 3-4 days to cure conjunctivitis.

15. **Excessive bleeding from wounds:** Dried cow dung is applied over the wound to control excessive bleeding.

16. **Sprains:**
    - *'Badha'* of *'Reja'* is crushed and the mixture is applied on the affected area.
    - The bark of *'Chila'* is crushed and mixed with water. The paste is applied on the affected area.

17. **Bodyache or pain in the joints**: A paste made of boiled Country Borage (*'Gabhar-Patha')* is applied o the affected area for relief.

18. **Vomiting:**
    - *'Var'* or *'Laberi'* is crushed in water and the paste is mixed with honey and licked for relief.
    - Burnt peacock feather is mixed with honey and taken.

19. **Earache:**
    - Bone of Peacock's foot is scrubbed in water and this water is put drop wise into the ear.
    - Baking soda and Lemon juice are put into the ear.

20. **Stomachache due to gas:**
    - Stomach massage using Kerosene oil is done.
    - Water kept overnight in Copper utensils is consumed.

21. **Snake/lizard bite**: Heated coin is kept on the bitten area to provide relief.

22. **Swelling:**
    - Massage is done using heated Mustard oil mixed with salt.
    - Indian Flame Tree *('Palash')* or *'Vesram'* is heated and tied on the affected area with a piece of cloth.

23. **On tumor formation:** 50 grams Jaggery and 25 grams Baking Soda is made into a paste and applied over the tumor. Hot compression is also given after the paste is applied.

24. **Vomiting in children**: Lemon juice, salt and sugar are mixed in a glass of water and given twice a day for relief.

25. Mouth ulcers: • Almonds (*'Chiraunji'*) are scrubbed and crushed in water and the paste is applied over the ulcer. • Leaves of Common Jasmine (*'Chameli'*) are chewed on to cure ulcers. • Black catechu *('Kattha')* is crushed and applied.
26. Boils on the body: The fruit of *'Rekha'* is burnt and the ash is mixed with pure *'Ghee'* and applied on the affected area.
27. Cold and cough: • Small Pepper *('Choti Pippali')* is crushed and mixed with honey and taken or the powder is mixed with jaggery and licked. Turmeric and sugar are dry roasted and mixed in honey. This preparation is licked on to cure cold and cough. • Turmeric, Pepper Longum *('Badi Pippali')*, Dry Ginger (*'Saunth'*) and Jaggery are boiled together in milk and taken. Drinking water is avoided for a while after drinking the above concoction.
28. Pneumonia or cough and cold in children: • 2-3 drops of Cow's urine is given to the child 3-4 times in a day. • The child is massaged with Cow's urine too.
29. Stomach-ache or cough and cold in children: • Asafoetida (*'Hing')* is heated and given along with milk. • The child is massaged using the same too.
30. Itching: • Cow's urine is applied over the affected area. The area is covered using fresh cow dung and sun-dried. After this a bath is taken. This procedure is repeated 2-3 times to get rid of itching. • Crushed Bush Tomato (*'Bhataktaiyya')* is mixed in water and strained. This extract is taken on an empty stomach to cure itching.

Dosage: 1 spoonful for children and 2-3 spoonfuls for adults. 2-3 red chillies are heated in mustard oil and the oil is applied over the affected area.
31. **To prevent Hair fall:** A paste made of crushed Trailing Eclipta (*'Ghamra'*) leaves is applied on the hair and scalp and sun-dried. It is then rinsed off. The procedure is repeated twice a day to cure hair fall problems.
32. **Acne/Warts:** • Juice of leaves of Cashew Nut (*'Chirol'*) applied on Acne/Warts. • Hairs from tail of horse massaged at the site of Warts and then they cut
33. **Sore throat:** • Salt mixed in lukewarm water is used for gargling. • Black tea made of Carom seeds (*'Ajwain'*) is taken. • Joint made of Carom seeds (*'Ajwain'*) is smoked.
34. **Treatment of Aav:** • Drink made up of pulp of Bael fruit (*'Bel'*) used. • Leaves of Jambol (*'Jamun'*), seeds of Jambol (*'Jamun'*), tender leaves of Margosa (*'Neem'*) and Rice Plant (*'Vihi'*), Carom seeds (*'Ajwain'*), Black salt crushed together to make tablets. 3 tablets given twice or thrice a day.
35. **Dhat (Leucorrhoea):** • Powder of seeds of Jambol (*'Jamun'*) taken empty stomach with water. • *Pulp* of fruit of Indian Flame Tree (*'Palash'*) crushed with honey and taken 3-4 times a day is beneficial. • Spreading Hogweed (*Chat of 'Patthar'*) crushed in water given orally.
36. **Jaundice:** • Sugarcane juice (*'Ekshu Rasa'*) and *'Papaya'* are consumed. • Certain magico-cultural rituals are also followed.
37. **Scorpion bite:** • Crushed leaves of *'Adde jhaare'* are applied over the bitten area. • A small electric current is passed through the body to provide relief from the pain of scorpion bite.

• Certain magico-cultural rituals are also followed. • The effect of scorpion bite is reduced with faecal matter of elephant. • Cloves, Sulphur, Iron Salt and Indian Mustard etc. tied together in cloth used to cure the bite effects with *Mantra*. • Feather of Peacock is used with *Mantra*.
38. **Burns:** Salt water or raw Potato is applied over the burnt area.
39. **For strengthening and blackening of hair:** A hair pack made of Black Soil, Lemon and Buttermilk is applied and rinsed off on drying.
40. **Fever:** • Tea made of Holy Basil (*'Tulsi'*) leaves and seeds is taken. • Vegetable dish made of fresh leaves of Sickel Senna (*'Puar'*) eaten for sweating. After sweating the fever reduces. • A decoction made of Margosa (*'Neem'*) leaves is taken. • Roots of Tinospora (*'Gurbel'*) is crushed and taken along with milk.
41. **Maria Fever:** *'Sanjeevani Tablet'* + Stem of Tinospora (*'Guruvej'*) crushed with honey and taken orally.
42. **For Typhoid Fever (*'Motijhara'*):** *'Sanjeevani'* herb and ashes of pearls is taken.
43. **Thorn prick:** • Extract of Aloe Vera (*'Pauhra'*) is applied to provide relief. • Crushed *'Bhata'* is applied over the affected area. The thorn comes out on doing this.
44. **Bodyache due to gas formation:** Asafoetida (*'Hing'*) is heated and taken.
45. **Tongue burn:** Black salt is consumed to provide relief.
46. **Gas formation:** Black salt, Cumin seeds (*'Jeera'*), dry Coriander, Cardamom, Black Pepper and Fennel seeds

(*'Saunph'*) are mixed and crushed together and taken to provide relief.

47. Indigestion: Buttermilk mixed with black salt is taken.

48. After Delivery:

- After Delivery water boiled with Margosa tree (*'Neem'*) leaves used for bathing purposes by mothers.
- Water boiled with Margosa *('Neem')* leaves, bark of Black Catechu (*'Khair'*), Carom Seeds (*'Ajwain'*) etc. boiled in water. After cooling, this water is given to mother twice a day. This is beneficial in post partum period.
- Carom seeds *('Ajwain')* is burnt to form smoke. This smoke is given to mother and child.
- Children are given mixture of paste of Almond, Nutmeg (*'Jaiphal'*), paste of 'Aethani', Borax *('Suhaga')*, Turmeric powder (*'Haldi'*), Saffron *('Kesar')*.
- Mothers are given *'Harira'* up to one year after delivery. *'Harira'* made by mixing Jaggery, dry fruits, *Ghee*, Carom seeds *('Ajwain')*, Dry Ginger, Pepper *('Pippali')* to make a mixture. This mixture is mixed with milk and milk is boiled. After cooling this milk is given to mother.
- Turmeric powder (*'Haldi'*), Dry Fruits fried in *Ghee* and mixed with Lin seeds *('Alsi')* to form *Laddu*. These Laddus are beneficial in post partum period.

49. Headache:

- A paste made of crushed Mustard seeds is applied.
- A paste made of crushed Eucalyptus leaves and water is applied.
- Peppermint or camphor is added to coconut oil and this oil is applied.

50. Stomachache and other gastric problems: Water kept overnight in Copper utensil is consumed.

51. To promote mental strength: 50gms Jaggery is taken every night before going to bed.

52. For clear bowels: A glassful of water is taken before going for the bowels. This promotes a clear stomach.

53. **Massage to Children:**
    - *'Lal' Tel* is used.
    - Mustard *('Rai)'*, Garlic, Fenugreek *('Methi')*, Carom Seeds, Asafoetida *('Hing')* boiled in Mustard oil. This oiled is used for massaging of mothers and children. For mothers it can be used for 15-20 days after delivery and for children it can be used for 1.5-2 months.

54. **Cough/Kukur Khansi:**
    - *Pulp ('Gad')* of India Flame Tree *('Palash')* crushed and then mixed with Honey and taken orally.
    - Peacock feather burnt to make ashes and mixed with honey to be taken orally.
    - Ginger, Garlic paste mixed with Honey and given orally frequently.

55. **Excessive menstrual bleeding:** A decoction made of crushed Cumin Seeds *('Jeera)* and sugar in water is taken.

56. **Cold:** One of the types of Cactus or Milk Bush *('Nagpheni')* crushed with water and given orally.

57. **Irregular menstrual cycle:** Flowers of Thatch Grass *('Kaans')* are burnt and mixed with honey and taken to regularize menstrual cycles.

58. **Avoiding Mosquito Bites:**
    - Fumigation by Sulphur.
    - Kerosene Oil *('Mitti ka Tel')* applied on skin
    - Cow dung and Sickel Senna *('Puar')* burnt to form smoke

59. **Boil:**
    - Seed of Sickel Senna *('Puar')* grinded to make paste. The paste is applied locally.
    - Leaves of Gourd are crushed and applied on the boils to cure them.

60. **For sobering up of the alcohol addiction:** Drinking juice of Lemon is beneficial.

61. **For early Eruption of Teeth:** Gums massaged with Honey.

62. **Oedema:** Leaves of *'Vesram'* are heated and applied on affected part
63. **To promote lactation:** • Porridge made of *'Dalia'* and raw Papaya is given. • Powdered Common Bur (*'Kadam'*) flowers are given along with milk to promote lactation.
64. **Insomnia:** Goat's milk is massaged onto the hands and feet to promote good sleep.
65. **Wounds:** Burnt Turmeric is mixed with Mustard oil and applied on the wound.
66. **Jaundice:** A vegetable dish made of raw Papaya is taken. Chillies are not added to this preparation.
67. **Dog bite:** Extract of Madar (*'Auk'*) is applied. Certain magico-cultural rituals are also followed.
68. **Wounds:** Alum and a pinch of salt is added to a cup of water and applied over the wound to control bleeding.
69. **Fracture:** • Leaves of Five Leave Chaste (*'Nirgudi)* are tied over the fractured area. • Leaves of the Five Leave Chaste (*'Nirgudi)* are crushed and taken along with water.
70. **Wounds:** Leaves of Trailing Eclipta (*'Ghamra'*) is burnt and applied over the wounds to cure it.
71. **To promote lactation:** White Bermuda Grass (*'Duva'*) is crushed and taken 2-3 times in a day along with milk to promote lactation.
72. **Vomiting:** *'Lakheri'* and Cardamom is taken.
73. **Worms in the stomach:** False Black Pepper (*'Vaividanga'*) is crushed and taken along with milk to get relief.

Annexure 3(c)

Medicinal Plant Names—Madhya Pradesh

Vernacular Name	*English Name*	*Sanskrit Name*	*Botanical Name*
Aak	Madar	*Ark*	*Calotropis procera*
Aam	Mango	*Amratak*	*Mangifera indica*
Aphu	Opium	*Ahiphen*	*Papaver somniferum*
Ajwain	Carom Seeds	*Ajmoda*	*Carum roxburghianum*
Alsi	Lin Seed/Flax Seeds	*Alsi*	*Linum usitassimum*
Alu	Potato	*Aluk*	*Solanum tuberosum*
Amrud	Guava		
Anar	Pomegranate	*Dadim*	*Punica granatum*
Andi	Castor Oil Plant	*Aerand Karkati*	*Ricinus comunis*

Vernacular Name	*English Name*	*Sanskrit Name*	*Botanical Name*
Awala/Amla	Indian Gooseberry	*Amalaki*	*Embelica officinalis*
Babul	*Babul*	*Kinkirak*	*Acacia arabica*
Bach	Sweat Flag Root	*Vacha*	*Acorus calamus*
Badi Elayachi	Big Cardamom	*Vela*	*Amommum sublatum*
Bel	Bael	*Bilva/Shriphal*	*Aegele marmelos*
Bhataktaiyya	Bush Tomato/India Night shade	*Bruhati*	*Solanum indicum*
Bhilma	Making Nut	*Bhallatak*	*Semecarpus anacardium*
Chameli	Common Jasmine	*Jati*	*Jasmine officinale*
Chandan	Sandal	*Rakta Chandan*	*Ptero Carpus satalinus*
Chiraul	Chiraunji Nut Tree	*Priyal/Char*	*Buchania lanzan*
Chiraunji	Almond	*Vatam*	*Prunus dulcis*
Chirol	Cashew Nut	*Agnikrit/Kajutak*	*Holoptela in tegrifola*
Chat of Pathhar	Spreading Hogweed	*Punarnava*	*Boerhavia diffusa*
Dhaniya	Dry Coriander	*Dhyanyak*	*Coriandrum sativum*
Dudhghass	Asthma Plant	*Chara*	*Euphorbia hirta*
Duva	Burmuda Grass	*Durva*	*Cunodon dacrylon*
Emali	Tamarind	*Amlika/Tintandik*	*Tamarindus indica*
Elayachi	Cardamom	*Aela*	*Elettaria cardmoum*
Engua	Desert Date/Soap Berry Tree	*Engudi*	*Balnites aegyptiaca*

Vernacular Name	*English Name*	*Sanskrit Name*	*Botanical Name*
Gabhar-Patha	Country Borage	*Pashan Bhed*	*Coleus aromaticus*
Gajar	Carrot	*Garjaram*	*Daucus carota*
Ganna	Sugarcane	*Ekshwaku*	*Saccharum officinarum*
Gavar Patha	Aloe Vera	*Ghrit Kumari*	*Aloe barbadensis*
Genda	Marigold	*Zanduk*	*Tagetus erecta*
Ghamra	Trailing Eclipta	*Brungraj*	*Eclipta alba*
Gulab	Rose	*Taruni*	*Rosa centifolia*
Gunja	Indian Liquorice	*Gunja*	*Abrus precatorius*
Guruvej	Tinospora	*Giloy*	*Tinospora cordifolia*
Hadjod	Veld Grape	*Asthi Samharak*	*Cissus quadrangularis*
Haldi	Turmeric	*Haridra*	*Curcuma longa*
Hing	Asafoetida	*Hing*	*Ferula assfoetida*
Jaiphal	Nutmeg	*Jatiphal*	*Myristica fragrance*
Jamun	Jambol	*Jambu*	*Syzygium cumim*
Kadam	Common Bur	*Kadamb*	*Anthocephalus cadamba*
Kaiphal/Aar	Box Myrtle/Bayberry	*Kaiphal*	*Myrica nagi*
Kandi	Sponge tree	*Shami*	*Prosopis cineramia specigera*
Kanko	Tailed Pepper/Cubeb/Java Pepper	*Kankol*	*Piper cubeba*

Vernacular Name	*English Name*	*Sanskrit Name*	*Botanical Name*
Kans	Thatch Grass	*Kash*	*Saccharum spontaneum*
Kesar	Saffron	*Kukumam*	*Crocus sativus*
Kev	Fragrant Screw Pine	*Ketaki*	*Pandramus odortiomis*
Khair/Kattha	Black Catechu	*Gayatri*	*Acacia catechu*
Koha	Arjun	*Arjun*	*Termnalia arjuna*
Kali Mirch	Black Pepper	*Marich*	*Piper nigrum*
Lahsun	Garlic	*Rason*	*Allium sativum*
Lavang	Clove	*Devkusum/ Shriprasun*	*Syzygium aromaticum*
Mahua	Butter Tree	*Madhu Pushpak*	*Madhuka longifolia*
Mehndi	Henna	*Madayantica*	*Lowsonia inermis*
Methi	Fenugreek	*Methika*	*Trigonalla faenugraecum*
Mirch	Red Chilly	*Katuvira*	*Capsicum annum*
Nagpheni/ Thuhar	Milk Bush/Cactus	*Snuhi*	*Euphorbia nerifolia*
Neem	Margosa	*Nimb*	*Azadirecta indica*
Nilgiri	Eucalyptus		
Nimbu	Lemon	*Nimbuk*	*Citrus aurantifolia*
Nirgundi	Five Leaved Chask	*Nirgundi/Sindurvar*	*Vitex nigundo*

Vernacular Name	English Name	Sanskrit Name	Botanical Name
Palash	Flame of Forest	*Palash*	Butea monosperma
Papaya	Papaya	*Aerandkarkati*	*Carica papaya*
Patharcha	Spreading Hogweed	*Punarnava*	*Boerhavia diffusa*
Pipal	Peepal	*Ashwath*	*Ficus religiosa*
Pippali	Long Pepper	*Pippali*	*Piper longum*
Pudina	Mint	*Putiha*	*Memtha spicate*
Puar/Puvar	Sickel Senna	*Chakramard*	*Cassia tora*
Pyas	Onion	*Palandu*	*Allium cepa*
Rai	Mustard	*Rajika*	*Brassica juncea*
Satavar	Asparagus	*Shatavari*	*Asparagus racemosus*
Saunph	Fennel Seeds	*Mishreya*	*Foeniculum vulgare*
Semar	Silk Cotton Tree	*Shalmali*	*Bombax ceiba*
Supari	Betel	*Poog*	*Areca catechu*
Tinsa	Sandal Chariot	*Tinasha/Syandan*	*Ougenia oojeinensis*
Tulsi	Holy Basil	*Tulsi*	*Ocimum sactum*
Vaiding	False Black Pepper	*Vidang*	*Embelica ribes*
Vihi	Rice Plant	*Vrihi*	*Oryza sativa*

Annexure 4(a)

Home Remedies, Bilaspur District—Chhattisgarh

RESPIRATORY SYSTEM

Cough and Cold

Sl. No.	*Name of Medicinal Plant*	*Method of Preparation*
1.	Holy Basil + Ginger + Turmeric Powder	Holy Basil + Ginger crushed together and Turmeric added and given orally.
2.	Turmeric Powder + *'Kanaki Chaswal Atta'*	—
3.	*'Harri Zor'* + Red Chili + Turmeric Powder	*'Harri Zor'* + Red Chilli + Turmeric Powder mixed together and given.
4	Holy Basil + Honey	Holy Basil crushed with Honey.
5.	*'Karil'* + Turmeric Powder + Black Pepper *('Kali Mirch')*	*'Karil'* + Turmeric Powder + Black Pepper *('Kali Mirch')* mixed together and taken.
6.	Ginger +Holy Basil + Eucalyptus + Black Pepper *('Kali Mirch')*	Ginger +Holy Basil + Eucalyptus crushed together and *Kali Mirch* added to mixture and given orally.

Sl. No.	Name of Medicinal Plant	Method of Preparation
7.	Cloves of Garlic + *'Ghee'* (Clarified Butter)	Garlic Cloves are fries in *Ghee* and given.
8.	Outer covering of bark of *'Dahiman'* + Sweat flag root	Powder of outer covering of bark of *'Dahiman'* + Sweat flag root mixed together and given.
9.	Chebulic Myrobalan (*'Hirra'*) + Beleric Myrobalam (*'Behda'*) or young Chebulic Myrobalan (*'Hirara'*)	*'Hirda'* and *'Behda'* are fried and then crushed to make powder. Powder is taken orally.
10.	Dry Ginger, Cloves + Black Pepper (*Kali Mirch*) + Long Pepper	Dry Ginger + Cloves + Black Pepper (*Kali Mirch*) + Long Pepper crushed and added in water with salt and then water is heated and it is used as drink.
11.	Ginger + Holy Basil Leaves + Turmeric Powder	Ginger + Holy Basil Leaves + Turmeric Powder added to normal tea and taken.

Other plants mentioned by villagers are leaves of Eucalyptus, Asafetida, Fenugreek seeds, Mustard oil, *'Bhatkattaiya'*, *'Kulangan'*, Honey, *'Bach Kanda'*, Vapours of Water.

DIGESTIVE SYSTEM

Gas

Sl. No.	Name of Medicinal Plant	Method of Preparation
1.	'Bagdol Kanda' (Onion) + Alcohol made from Butter Tree ('Mahua')	Crushed 'Bagdol Kanda' added to 'Mahua' and use as a drink.

Pain in Abdomen

Sl. No.	*Name of Medicinal Plant*	*Method of Preparation*
1.	Outer covering of bark of *'Dahiman'* + Alcohol made from Butter Tree (*'Mahua'*)	Outer covering of bark of *'Dahiman'* crushed in + Alcohol made from Butter Tree *('Mahua')*.
2.	Outer covering of bark of Mango Tree + Outer covering of bark of Babbul Tree + Outer covering of bark of Margosa Tree + fruit of Jambol	Outer covering of bark of Mango Tree + Outer covering of bark of Babbul Tree + Outer covering of bark of Margosa Tree + fruit of Jambol are crushed to make juice and the juice is taken.
3.	Oil of Mustard + Salt	Local application of Oil of Mustard + Salt.

Diarrhoea

Sl. No.	*Name of Medicinal Plant*	*Method of Preparation*
1.	Root of *'Sindhadi'*	Root of *'Sindhadi'* crushed in water and given.
2.	Outer covering of bark of Mango and *'Kosal'* Tree	Outer covering of bark of Mango and *'Kosal'* Tree crushed in water and given orally.
3.	Root of *'Gengrava'*	Root of *'Gengrava'* crushed in water and given.
4.	Old dried Mango powder (*'Amchur'*) + Lemon water	Old dried Mango powder (*'Amchur'*) taken with Lemon water.
5.	*'Saphed Musali'* (Asparagus) + Leaves of Gaub Tree *('Tendupatta')*	*'Saphed Musali'* + Leaves of Gaub Tree *('Tendupatta')* are chewed.

Sl. No.	Name of Medicinal Plant	Method of Preparation
6.	Fruit of *'Sarai'* + Salt	Fruit of *'Sarai'* crushed and taken with Salt

Constipation

Names mentioned by villagers of home remedies of Constipation are Chebulic Myrobalan (*'Hirra'*), *'Triphala'* (Powder of dry fruits of Chebulic Myrobalan, Beleric Myrobalam and Indian Gooseberry), *'Amchur'*, Aloe Vera, Turmeric Powder, Asafoetida, Pepper, Black Salt, *'Gohinja'*, Outer covering of bark of *'Babbul'* and *'Dahiman'*, Alcohol made up of Indian Butter Tree (*'Mahua)'*, *'Bagdol Kand'*, Leaves of *'Bijata'*, *'Lagvanti'*.

Vomiting

Names mentioned by villagers of home remedies of vomiting are Leaves of *'Devana'*, Onion, Honey and Mint Leaves.

Diarrhoea

Names mentioned by villagers of home remedies of diarrhoea are salt, sugar, lemon, *'Dashman'* flower, tea powder, outer covering of bark of *'Parasa'*, *'Phudaki'* and *'Sarai'*, Root of *'Dobi'*, *'Gengruva'*, Bael, *'Chuee Mitti'*, Leaves of *'Tendu'*, Eucalyptus tree, Asparagus, Dry Ginger, *'Gorakhmundi'*, *'Saphed Musali'*.

ENT

Earache

Sl. No.	Name of Medicinal Plant	Method of Preparation
1.	Margosa leaves	Margosa leaves boiled in water and the drops of water after cooling put into ear.

Toothache

Sl. No.	*Name of Medicinal Plant*	*Method of Preparation*
1.	Black Salt (*'Sendhav Namak'*) + Turmeric Powder + Mustard	Black Salt (*'Sendhav Namak'*)+ Turmeric Powder + Mustard heated and rubbed on teeths.
2.	Leaves of Mango tree	Leaves of Mango tree are boiled in water and filtered water is used for gargling purposes.

Names mentioned by villagers for home remedies of toothache are Fruit of *'Bhatkataiya'*, Flower of *'Gulmohar'*, Turmeric Powder, Mustard oil.

SKIN

Itching of Skin

Sl. No.	*Name of Medicinal Plant*	*Method of Preparation*
1.	Oil of *'Dori'*	Local application
2.	Oil of Coconut	Local application
3.	Leaves of Margosa	Paste of leaves of Margosa locally applied
4.	Oil of *'Karaj'* and *' Kosam'*	Local application

Names mentioned by villagers of home remedies for Skin Diseases are leaves of Tomato plant, Salt, Cow dung, *'Phundaraban'*, Sesame oil, Seed of *'Seetaphal'*, *Ajwain*, Carom Seeds.

GYNAECOLOGICAL COMPLAINTS

Lactogenic

Sl. No.	*Name of Medicinal Plant*	*Method of Preparation*
1.	Pepper	Crushed Pepper mixed with milk and given orally.

Black Gram, Raw Papaya, milk, Pipper, Extract of Banyan tree are also mentioned by villagers.

Weakness after Delivery

Sl. No.	*Name of Home Remedy*	*Method of Preparation*
1.	*'Hirva Chor'* + *'Rohina'* + *'Baba Jata'* + Cloves of Garlic	*'Hirva Chor', 'Rohina', 'Baba Jata',* cloves of Garlic boiled in milk and the milk is given orally.
2.	Cashew Nuts + Dry Ginger + Carom Seeds + Jaggery + Dates + *'Soham'* + Turmeric powder + *'Parag'* + *'Cattaiv'* + Asafoetida + Black Pepper + Coconut	*Laddu* made up of Cashew Nuts, Pepper, Dry Ginger, Carom Seeds, Jaggery, Dates, *Soham,* Turmeric powder, *Parag, Cattaiv,* Asafoetida, Black Pepper, Coconut given for 15 days to 1 month.

Pain during Menstruation

Sl. No.	*Name of Medicinal Plant*	*Method of Preparation*
1.	Cloves + Garlic + Black Salt	Paste of Cloves + Garlic + Black Salt is given.

Other medicinal plants mentioned by villagers are *'Hirva'* (*'Kulathi dal'*), Garlic, flower of *'Gudhal'*, leaves of *'Muli'*, (Sugar, water of washed rice).

For Easy Delivery

Mustard Oil, Warm Milk, Tea made up of Jaggery, Fresh warm *khichadi.*

Massage after Delivery

Mustard Oil, Asafetida, Carom seeds, Garlic, *'Charka Gomachi'.*

Post Partum Period Health Improvement

Dry fruits like Cashew Nuts, Almonds, Dry Dates, Dry Coconut, Dry Ginger, Pepper, Extract from *Babul* Tree, Jaggery, Clarified Butter, *'Chiraunji'.*

ACUTE CONDITIONS

Headache

Sl. No.	*Name of Medicinal Plant*	*Method of Preparation*
1.	Outer covering of bark of *'Chanhor'*	Outer covering of bark of *'Chanhor'.*
2.	Leaves of Thorn Apple tree (*'Dhatura'*)	Leaves of Thorn Apple (*'Dhatura'*) crushed to form paste is applied on head.

Other herbs mentioned by villagers are Garlic, Onion, Bitter Melon, Aloe Vera, leaves of Eucalyptus, leaves of Marigold plant, leaves of Bariyari plant, Outer covering of bark of Mango tree.

Fever

Sl. No.	Name of Medicinal Plant	Method of Preparation
1.	Sweat Chirette	Leaves of Sweat Chirette boiled in water and the filtered water taken orally or Sweat Chirette taken with warm water.
2.	*'Bhatkataiya'*	*'Bhatkataiya'* taken with warm water.
3.	Cordifolia	Root of Cordifolia with warm water.

Malaria

Sl. No.	Name of Medicinal Plant	Method of Preparation
1.	Leaves of Margosa + Bael + *'Gatarun'* + Root of *'Bhatkataiya'* + Cordifolia root + Black Pepper (*'Kali Mirch'*)	Leaves of Margosa' + Bael + *'Gatarun'* + Root of *'Bhatkataiya'* + Cordifolia root + *'Kali Mirch'* crushed and mixed with water and taken orally.
2.	Sweat Chirette	Leaves of Sweat Chirette crushed in boiled water taken orally.

Other plants mentioned by villagers are *'Bhuineemb'*, outer covering of bark of Mango tree, *'Chirchita'*.

Bone Fracture

Sl. No.	Name of Medicinal Plant	Method of Preparation
1.	Root of *'Asthisanharak'* + *'Kharha'* + *'Dasna'*	Powder of Root of *Asthisanharak, Kharha, Dasna* applied over affected area.

Other plants mentioned by villagers are outer covering of bark of '*Couraiya*' and '*Sarai*', *Kand of 'Amrola'*, '*Goinja*'.

MISCELLANEOUS

Joint Pain

Sl. No.	*Name of Medicinal Plant*	*Method of Preparation*
1.	'*Vanrakias Kanda*' + Mustard Oil	'*Vanrakias Kanda*' + Mustard Oil used for local application.

Other plants mentioned by villagers are Carom seeds, cloves of Garlic, Mustard oil, Outer covering of bark of '*Rohina*', Oil of '*Redi*', Asafoetida, '*Gomayi*', '*Balarakas*', '*Koriya*', '*Korja*'.

Jaundice

Sl. No.	*Name of Medicinal Plant*	*Method of Preparation*
1.	Drum stick	Leaves of Drum Steak are boiled in water and this water is used for bathing. And the decoction made by Drum Steak leaves taken orally.
2.	Dodder ('*Amar Vel*')	Leaves of Dodder ('*Amar Vel*') are boiled in water and this water is used for bathing. And the decoction made of '*Amar Vel*' leaves taken orally.

Wound

Sl. No.	*Name of Medicinal Plant*	*Method of Preparation*
1.	Ashes *('Rakh')* + Lime *('Chuna')*	Local application of Ashes ('Rakh') + Lime (*'Chuna'*).
2.	Kerosene	Local application of Kerosene.
3.	Outer covering of bark of Margosa tree	Powder of outer covering of bark of Margosa tree locally applied.
4.	Outer covering of bark of Margosa tree	
5.	*'Jatropha' (Ratanjyot, S. Darvanti*)	Extract from *'Jatropha'* applied on wound.

Other plants mentioned by villagers are *Goenja,* Turmeric powder, *Chuna,* Seed of *Karanj,* Oil of *Dori, Bhakenda,* Kerosene, extract of *Ratanjyot,* outer covering of bark of Saleha.

Stroke/Hemiplegia

Sl. No.	*Name of Medicinal Plant*	*Method of Preparation*
1.	Root of *'Khapra'*	Root of *'Khapra'* crushed in water and given orally.

Root of *Khapra* plant, meat of Pigeon bird are also mentioned by villagers.

Weakness

Sl. No.	*Name of Medicinal Plant*	*Method of Preparation*
1.	*'Hirva Zor'* and *'Arhar'* (Pigeon Pea) *'chhor'*	Drinking orally.

Other ingredients of home remedies mentioned by villagers are prons, Chick pea (*'chana'), kand* of *'Telia', 'Tejraj'*, roots of *'Bhojraj', 'Kamraj', 'Balaraj'*, Juice of Indian Butter Tree, White *'Gomayi'*, Jaggery, Potato, Clarified Butter, *'Phalli', 'Badrava kanda'*.

Kidney Stone

Outer covering of bark of *'Mahali'*.

Diabetes

Leaves of Margosa tree mentioned by villagers.

Dhat (STDs)

Outer covering of bark of Cauraiya and Dagdua tree.

Snake Bite

Saleha, Kalmi, outer covering of bark of Indian Butter Tree.

Piles

Lotus flower, Thorn Apple, alcohol made up from Indian Butter Tree.

Annexure 4(b)

Baiga Remedies, Bilaspur District—Chhattisgarh

MARWAHI BLOCK

Name of Disease	*Local name of disease*	*Plant used*		*Part used*	*Other Product used*	*Preparation*	*Doses*	*Duration/ Taboo*
		Local name	*Botanical name*					
1	2	3	4	5	6	7	8	9
1. Fever	Jar	*Gataran*	*Caesalpinia crista*	Fruit	Water	By grinding	One small cup twice a day	3 days
		Peeper	*Piper longum*	Fruit				
		Gataran	*Caesalpinia crista*	Seed, Leaf	Water	By grinding	One small cup twice a day	3 days
		Sonth	*Zingiber officinale*	Rhi-zome	Water		Two tea-spoon full,	2-3 days

1	2	3	4	5	6	7	8	9
		Peeper	*Piper longum*	Fruit			twice a day.	
		Laung		Fruit				
		Kali-mirch	*Piper Nigrum*	Fruit				
		Guruch	*Tinospora cordifolia*	Root	Water	By grinding	Two tea-spoon full, twice a day	3 days
2. Malaria	Thand-jur	*Bhatkattiya*	*Solanum indicum*	Root	Water	By grinding	One small cup twice a day	3 days
		Gataran	*Caesalpinia crista*	Fruit	Water	By boiling	One small cup twice a day	2-3 day
		Guruch	*Tinospora cordifolia*	Bark				
		Bhue Neem	*Phyllanthus niruri*	Leaf	Water	By grinding	One tea-spoon full, twice a day	3 days
		Neem	*Azadirecta indica*	Leaf	Water	By grinding	One small cup twice a day	3 days
		Bel	*Aegel marmelos*	Leaf				
		Gataran	*Caesalpinia crista*	Leaf				
		Guruch	*Tinospora cordifolia*	Steam				Rice

1	2	3	4	5	6	7	8	9
		Bhatkataiya	*Solanum indicum*	Fruit				
		Kali-Mirch	*Piper Nigrum*	Fruit				
		Ataria-ghadi		Root	Water	By grinding	One cup	3 day
		Malhin tree			Mustered oil	By grinding	—	3 day
		Hing	*Ferula assafoetida*	Gum				
		Gataran	*Caesalpinia crista*	Leaf	Water	By grinding	Every morning one cup per day.	3-4 days
		Neem	*Azadirecta indica*	Stem+ Leaf				
		Bel	*Aegel marmelos*	Stem+ Leaf				
		Kali-mirch	*Piper Nigrum*	Fruir				Sour, Chilli, *Urad* Pulse, Spices.
		Tulsi	*Ocimum sanctum*	Stem+ Leaf				
		Harsanghari	*Nictanthus arbortritis*	Leaves, Bark				
		Bhooi neem kalazira		Leaves	Jaggery and	Grinding and Making small	Two times in a day	3 days

1	2	3	4	5	6	7	8	9
		Banzeer		Seed	Honey	balls		Sour Fruit, Brinjal and Beans
		Gataran	*Caesalpinia crista*	Seed				
3. Jaundice Piri		*Dahiman*	*Cordia macleodi*	Bark	Water	By grinding	Two tea-spoon full, twice a day	7 days Oil and Chilli
		Guruch	*Tinospora cordifolia*	Root	Water	By grinding and Boiling.	Half cup twice a day	7 days
		Kirkich		Root				
		Pharhadda		Root				Turmeric, Oil and Chilli
		Gataran	*Caesalpinia crista*	Root				
		Charmuhi		Whole plant	Water	By grinding and mixing	One cup twice a day	3 days Sour food, Beans, Brinjal, Spice
		Dantul		Root	Water	By grinding	One tea-spoon full, twice a day	3 days Oily Foods
		Hingraj		Root	Water	By boiling	Bathing	3 day
		Amarbel	*Cuscuta reflexa*	Stem				

1	2	3	4	5	6	7	8	9
								Turmeric, Chilli and Oil
		Mango	*Mangifera indica*	Bark				
		Bahera	*Terminalia bellerica*	Fruit				
		Kosam	*Scheichera trigjuga*	Bark				
		Mahua	*Madhuka indica*	Bark				
		Neem	*Azadiecta indica*	Leaves				
		Saleha						
		Jamun	*Eugenia jambolana*	Bark				
		Mango	*Mangifera indica*	Bark	Water or Milk	By grinding	One cup per day	3 day
		Bahera	*Terminalia bellerica*	Bark				Turmeric, Spices and Oil
		Galgala	*Cochlospermum gossyium*	Bark				
		Ramband		Root	Water	By grinding	One cup per day	3 day
4. Bone-fracture		*Giloh*	*Tinospora Cordifolia*	Stem	Water	By grinding	One small cup twice a day	1 day.
	•	*Harsan-ghari*	*Nictanthus arbortritis*	Bark				

1	2	3	4	5	6	7	8	9
5.	Patha	*Peeper*	*Piper longum*	Root	Water	By grinding	One small cup twice a day	3 days
		Mahua	*Madhuka indica*	Root				
		Mango	*Mangifera indica*	Bark	Milk	By grinding	Two tea-spoon full, three times per day	7 days
		Jamun	*Syzygium cumin/Eugenia jambolana*	Bark				
		Dahiman	*Cordia macleodi*	Bark	Water	By grinding	Two tea-spoon full, three times per day	7 days Chilli and *Masala*
		Bhond		Root	Water	By grinding	Two tea-spoon full, three times per day	7 days
		Tinpatia	*Oxalis corniculata*	Root	Liquor	By grinding	One small cup twice a day	1 day
6. Piles	Babasur	*Koraiya*	*Holarrhena antidysentrica*	Bark	Liquor	By grinding and sitting them	Twice a day	3 months *Urad* pulse, Chilli and Brinjal
		Jimikand	*Amorphophallus campanulatus*	Tuber				
		Semar	*Bombax ceiba*	Tuber	-	By boiling	Twice a day	3 days Oily food.
		Ladies finger	*Abemoschus esculentus*	Fruit				

1	2	3	4	5	6	7	8	9
		Koraiya	*Holarrhena antidysentrica*	Bark	Jaggery	By grinding and made tablet form	Twice a day 2 tablets	3-4 days
		Dhatura	*Datura alba*	Fruit	Liquor	By mixing and sitting them	Twice a day	5 days
		Bokhla		Bark	Jaggery	By grinding, mixing and made tablet form	Twice a day 2 tablets.	21 days
		Balmusra		Bark	Jaggery	By grinding and made tablet form	One tablet per day	15/30 days
		Parsa		Tuber				Sour, Brinjal, *Udad*, pulse, Fish
		Bangondli		Tuber	Liquor	By grinding	One cup per day	3 days
		Saal	*Shorea robusta*	Bark				Sour foods
		Tilsa		Bark				
		Fagdul		Bark	Jagrey	By grinding and made tablet form	One tablet per day	8 days
		Korcott		Bark				Sour,

1	2	3	4	5	6	7	8	9
		Ajwain	*Carum roburghianum*	Fruit				Brinjal, *Udad* pulse
		Sonth	*Zinziber officinale*	Rhizome				
		Pepper	*Piper longum*	Fruit				
		Til	*Sesamum indicum*	oil	*Ghee*	By grinding	Apply in effected area	7 days Sour, Brinjal, *Udad* pulse
		Neela-thotha	*Copper Sulphate* *7CuSO₄.5 (H₂O)*					
		Black Dhatura		Leaf	Blood of pig and tortoise with pure Liquor	Grinding and obtain juice	Two times	One week Sour and spicy foods
7. Arthritis	Bat-rog	*Mainhar*		Tuber	Water	By boiling.	Twice a day one piece.	30 days.
		Sitka kanda		Tuber				
		Rawan-bitta		Root	Water	By grinding	Two tea-spoon full, twice a day	15 days
		Hathin		Leaf	–	By grinding and heating	Twice a day.	15 days
		Mahua	*Madhuka indica*	Flower				

1	2	3	4	5	6	7	8	9
		Indravan		Root	Castor (*Arandi*) oil	By boiling	Two times massage per day	30 days.
		Jhagarha		Tuber				
		Dhatura	*Datura alba*	Fruit				
		Gaanja	*Cannabis sativa*	Leaf				
		Aphim	*Papaver somniferum*	Leaf				
		Lavki	*Lagenaria scieraria*	Fruit				
		Scorpion		Animal				
		Singhrahri	*Trapa bi-spinosa*	Root	Water	By grinding	One small cup twice a day	8 days
8. Cough and Cold	—	*Pharha*		Bark	Water	By grinding	One tea-spoon full, twice a day	2 days
		Sonth,	*Zinziber officinale*	Rhi-zome	Water	By boiling	Two tea-spoon full, twice a day	3 days
		Kali Mirch	*Piper nigrum*	Fruit				
		Peeper	*Piper longum*	Fruit				
		Laung	*Syzygium aromaticum*	Fruit				
		Sonth,	*Zinziber officinale*	Rhizo me	Honey	By grinding and mixing.	Twice per day	3 days
		Piper	*Piper longum*	Fruit				

1	2	3	4	5	6	7	8	9
		Gomchi	*Abrus precatorius*	Fruit				
		Juice of pan	*Piper bitle*	Leaves				
9. Sto-mach pain	Pet-pira	*Bakayan kanda*	*Melia azadirecta*	Root	Water	By grinding	Three times per day.	2 days Liquor, Gaanja
		Dantul		Root	Water	By grinding	Half cup two or three times.	3 days
10. Itching pro-blem	Khajuri	*Kosam*	*Scheichera trigjuga*	Leaf	Water	By grinding	Two times massage per day	7 days
11. Weak-ness	-	*Ban kumhda*		Fruit	Honey	By grinding	One tea-spoon full, twice a day	15 days
12. Teeth pain	-	*Babool*	*Acacia Arabica*	Bark	-	By grinding	Bark attach to painful teeth	-
13.	Thanki	*Gingora*		Root	Water	By grinding	Two tea-spoon full, Twice a day	7 days
14. Head-ache		*Fundraban*		Flower	Water	By grinding	Two tea-spoons full.	1day.

1	2	3	4	5	6	7	8	9
15. *Dhaat*	–	*Bakayan kaanda*	*Melia azadirecta*	Root	Water and Sugar	By grinding	Two tea-spoon full, twice a day	15 days
		Kattilli		Root	Water	By grinding and made Chapati form	One chapati twice a day.	7 days
16. T.B.	Kapchae	–		–	Urine of goat and Copper coin	By boiling	Half cup twice a day	3 months oil and spices
		Sonth	*Zinziber officinale*	Rhi-zome	Jaggery	By grinding and Heating	One tablet every night.	3 months Sour, Brinjal
		Peeper, Ajwayan	*Piper longum Carum roxburghianum*	Fruit				
		Kali-Mirch	*Piper nigrum*	Fruit				
		Asgandh,	*Withania somnifera*	Fruit				
		Tejraj						
17. White dis-	–	*Akwan*	*Calotropis procera*	Root	Water	By grinding	Two tea-spoon full, twice a day	7 days

1	2	3	4	5	6	7	8	9
charge		*Kansi*		Root	Water	By grinding	Two tea-spoon full, twice a day.	7 days
		Patwan		Root	Water	By grinding	Half cup two or three times	3 days
18. Body heat		*Cactus*		Root	Water + Sugar	By grinding	Two tea-spoon full, twice a day	3 days
19. Cancer –		*Akwan*	*Calotropis gigantean*	Root	Water	By grinding	One tea-spoon full, twice a day	3 days
20.	Paath	*Guruch*	*Tinospora crdifolia*	Steam	Liquor	By grinding	One tea-spoon full, twice a day	3 days
		Chipphi		Root	Water	By grinding	Two teaspoon per day	5 day
21. Paraly-sis	Lakwa	*Sonth*	*Zinngiber officinale*	Rhizo-me	Milk	By grinding	One tablet twice a day	21 days Sour, Brinjal, Kumhda
		Dry fruits		Fruit				
		Piper	*Piper longum*	Fruit				
		Ajwain	*Carum roxburghianum*	Fruit				
		Saphed Moosli	*Chlorophytum tuberosum*	Root				

1	2	3	4	5	6	7	8	9
		Mirch,	*Capsicum annum*	Fruit				
		Asgandh, Tejraj.	*Withania somnifera*	Fruit				
		Chitavar	*Plumbago zeylanica*	Root	Water	By grinding	One small cup twice a day	15 days
		Satavar	*Asparagus racemosus*	Root	Pigeon Meat	By Boiling	–	3 days
		Jhagra		Flower	Mustered oil	By Boiling	Body massage two times per day	1 month
		Hing,	*Ferula asafetida*	Fruit				
		Lahsun	*Allium sativum*	Bulb				
		Nurani oil		-				
22. Filaria		*Korraiya*	*Holarrhena antidysentrica*	Bark	Water	By grinding	One small cup twice a day	1 month Sour
23. Snake bitting		*Katak*		Root	Water	By grinding	Half cup two or three times	1 day
		Chanahur		Root	Water	By grinding	Half cup two or three times	1 day
24. Cold-fever	Thand-jur	*Batilha*		Root	Water and Ginger	By Boiling	Two tea-spoon full, twice a day	4 days
		Gomchi	*Abrus precatorius*					

1	2	3	4	5	6	7	8	9
		Sonth	*Zinziber officinale*	Rhizome	juice.			
		Peeper	*Piper longum*	Fruit				
		Chiraita	*Swertia Chiraiyta*	Whole plant				
25. After delivery for health recovery		*Muthi*		Bark	Iron object	By grinding and heating with iron object.	Half cup twice a day	3 days
26. Lactation		*Khondu*		Bark	Water	By grinding	Half cup twice a day	2 days
		Mahua	*Madhuka indica*	Root				
27. Pain after delivery	Chewariya pira	*Mango*	*Mangifera indica*	Bark	Water	By boiling. Drink half cup and other used to take a bath to bath	Half cup twice a day	3 days
		Mahua	*Madhuka indica*	Flowers				
		Bel	*Aegel marmelos*	Bark				
		Jamun	*Eugania jambolana*	Bark				
		Mudhi.						
28. Menstrual Disturbance		*Gaingarua*	*Hibiscus sabdariffa*	Root	Liquor	By grinding	Half cup twice a day.	3 days
		Chula Dhavai		Flower				

1	2	3	4	5	6	7	8	9
		Bhue Dhumar	*Woodfordia fruticosa*	Fruit	Honey	By grinding and mixing.	Two tablets two times per day	3 days
		Saal	*Shorea robusta*	Stone	Sugar or Liquor or Jaggery or water	By grinding	Every morning one cup per day	3-4 days Sour, Chilli, *Udad* pulse, Spices
		Kosam	*Scheichera trijunga*	Bark				
		Bhogray		Root				
		Bam		Bark				
		Baherra	*Terminalia bellerica*	Bark				
		Dengarua		Bark				
		Ber	*Ziziphus jujuba*	Bark				
		Katri		Bark				
		Ainthi		Bark				
		Gud-sankri		Root				
		Kurlu		Root and Bark				
		Patthar-chatni		Fruit				
		Chandva		Root				
		Koljamras		Bark				
		Bamri		Root				

1	2	3	4	5	6	7	8	9
		Rakatvirar		Bark				
		Bemchi		Bark				
		Saphed gomchi		Seed				
		Masan jari		Root				
		Dhawai or Salya	*Woodfordia fruticosa*	Rhizo-me	Water	By grinding	Every morning one cup per day	1 days
		Dhania	*Cooriander sativum*	Seed	Water	By grinding	One cup per day	3 days
		Kashyap		Bark	Milk	By grinding	One cup per day	3 days
		Sher		Root	Liquor/ water	By grinding	One teaspoon twice a day	3-5 days Sour, *Udad* pulse
		Makra		Root				
		Pharhadda		Bark	Sugar and water	By grinding	One cup per day	3 days
29.	Kamal vaat	*Bagdol*		Fruit	Cow *Ghee*	By heating	Twice per day	3 days
30. Dirr-hoea		*Mango tree*		Bark	Water	By grinding and mixing	15 ml.	3 days Sour foods

1	2	3	4	5	6	7	8	9
31. Loose motion		*Ber tree*	*Ziziphus jujuba*	Leaves	Water	By grinding	1/2 cup	2 days
32. Skin disease		*Bhatkat-taiya*	*Solanum indicum*	Whole plant	Mustard oil	By grinding and mixing.	Apply in affected areas.	Till healing Sour foods.
33. Fever/ malaria	Jar-bukhar	*Bhatkat-taiya*	*Solanum indicum*	Root/ some time whole plant	water	By grinding and mixing.	1 cup	3 days Sour food, Beans
		Bhatkat-taiya *Gataran*	*Solanum indicum* *Caecalpinia crista*	Root, Seed	Water	By grinding and mixing	1 cup	3 days Sour food, Beans, Brinjal
34. Jhatka rog		*Taiti*		Root	Water	By grinding and mixing	1 cup	1 day
35. Intes-tine swel-ling	Patha	*Madar*	*Calotropis gigantean*	Leaves	–	By grinding	1 cup	3 days
		Phang		Root	Liquor	By grinding	One cup per day	3 day
		Dahiman	*Cordia macleodi*	Bark				
		Kharhad		Root	Water	By grinding	One cup per day	3 day

1	2	3	4	5	6	7	8	9
		Sendha		Leaves				
		Katai	*Jatropa curcas*	Tuber	Jaggery	By grinding and made tablet form	One tablet per day.	3 day
36. White-discharge	*Dhaat*	*Bhalmusri*		Bark	Water	By grinding and mixing	1 cup twice	one week Chilli, spice, oil and Sour foods
		Kursi		Root	-	By grinding and mixing	1 cup twice	3 days Sour foods, Chilli
		Korreya	*Holarhhena antidysentrica*	Bark				
		Tortoise		Meat	Oil and Water.	By heating	One cup per day	3 days Sour, Brinjal, *Udad* pulse
		Indravan		Root				
		Dahiman,	*Cordia macleodi*	Bark	Water/ Liquor	By heating	One cup per day	3 days
		Rohina and		Bark				
		Kakodohar		Bark				
		Mainhar		Root	Water	By grinding	One teaspoon twice a day	Till healing Sour foods
		Khadhari		Root				

1	2	3	4	5	6	7	8	9
		Fagdul		Root				
		Saal	*Shorea robusta*	Root				
37. Stone	Pathri	*Bokra kaanta*		Root	—	By grinding and mixing.	1/2 cup twice	One week
		Mango	*Mangifera indica*	Fruit				Chilli, Spice, oil and sour foods.
		Singrahani		Root	—	By grinding and mixing	1 cup	One week
38. Anal prob-lems	Guda rog	*Singrahani*		Root	—	By grinding and mixing	1 cup	3 days
		Akol	*Alangium lamarckii*	Root				Chilli, spice, oil and sour foods
39. T.B.		*Madar*	*Calotropis procera*	Leaves	Water	By grinding and mixing	1 cup	Till healing Chilli, spice, oil and Sour foods

1	2	3	4	5	6	7	8	9
40. Bone breaking		*Harsan-ghari*	*Nictanthus arbortritis*	Whole plant	Water	By grinding and mixing	Apply in affected areas	15 days *Udad* pulse, Beans Sour foods
		Khasna Dasna		Root	–	By grinding	Apply in affected areas	One day Spice, chilli
41. Head-ach	Mur-pira	*Daktarai*		Leaves	–	By grinding	Apply in forehead	One day
42. Snake, Scorpion and Dog bitting		*Jamrasi*		Bark	–	By grinding	Apply in affected area	Two times in one day Sour foods
43. Sujaak	–	*Balmusra* *Parsa,* *Bevri*		Root Tuber Tuber	Jaggery	By grinding and made tablet form	One tablet per day	15/30 days Sour, Brinjal, *Udad* pulse
		Sesume		Node	Water and Sugar	By grinding	One cup per day	3 days

Pendra Block

Name of Disease	Local name of disease	Plant used		Part used	Other Product used	Preparation	Doses	Duration/Taboo
		Local name	Botonical name					
1	2	3	4	5	6	7	8	9
1. Piles	Bavasir	*Balmusra*		Bark	Jagrey	By grinding and made tablet form	One tablet per day	15/30 days Sour, Brinjal, *Udad* pulse, Fish
		Parsa		Tuber				
		Bangondli		Tuber	Liquor	By grinding	One cup per day	3 days
		Saal	*Shorea robusta*	Bark				
		Tilsa	*Ougenia oojeinensis*	Bark				Sour foods
		Fagdul		Bark		By grinding and made tablet form	One tablet per day	8 days
		Korcott		Bark	Jaggery			
		Ajwayan,	*Carum roxburghianum*	Fruit				Sour, Brinjal, *Udad* pulse
		Sonth	*Zinngiber officinale*	Rhizome				
		Piper	*Piper longum*	Fruit				

1	2	3	4	5	6	7	8	9
		Til	*Sesamum indicum*	oil	*Ghee*	By grinding	Apply in effected area	7 days Sour, Brinjal, *Udad* Pulse
		Neela-thotha	*Copper Sulphate* 7$CuSO_4$.5 (H_2O)	-				
		Black Dhatura	*Datura stramonium*	Leaf	Blood of pig and tortoise with pure Liquor	Grinding and obtain juice	Two times	One week Sour and spicy foods
2. Sujaak	—	*Balmusra*		Root	Jagrey	By grinding and made tablet form	One tablet per day	15/30 days
		Parsa,		Tuber				
		Bevri		Tuber				Sour, Brinjal, *Udad* pulse.
		Sesum		Node	Water and Sugar	By grinding	One cup per day	3 days
3. White discharge	*Dhaat*	*Tortoise*		Meat	Oil and Water	By heating	One cup per day	3 days
		Indravan		Root				Sour, Brinjal, *Udad* Pulse
		Dahiman	*Cordia macleodi*	Bark	Water/	By heating	One cup	3 days

1	2	3	4	5	6	7	8	9
		Rohina		Bark	Liquor		per day	
		Kakodohar		Bark				
		Mainhar		Root	Water	By grinding	One teaspoon twice a day	Till healing Sour foods
		Khadhari		Root				
		Phagdul		Root				
		Saal	*Shorea robusta*	Root				
4.	*Paatha*	*Phang*		Root	Liquor	By grinding	One cup per day	3 days
		Dahiman	*Cordia macleodi*	Bark				
		Kharhad		Root	Water	By grinding	One cup per day	3 days
		Sendha		Leaves				
		Katai		Tuber	Jaggery	By grinding and made tablet form	One tablet per day	3 days
5. Jaundice	*Pilia*	*Hingraj*		Root	Water	By boiling	Bathing	3 days
		Amarbel	*Cuscuta reflexa*	Stem				
		Mango	*Mangifera indica*	Bark				Turmeric, Chilli and Oil
		Kosam	*Scheichera trijuga*	Bark				
		Neem	*Azadirecta*	Leaves				

1	2	3	4	5	6	7	8	9
			indica					
		Bahera	*Terminalia bellerica*	Fruit				
		Mahua	*Madhuka indica*	Bark				
		Saleha		Bark				
		Jamun	*Syzygium cumin/Eugenia jambolana*	Fruit Bark Seed				
		Mango	*Mangifera indica*	Bark	Water or Milk	By grinding	One cup per day	3 days
		Bahera	*Terminalia bellerica*	Bark				Turmeric, Spices Oil
		Galgala	*Chlorospermum gossypium*	Bark				
		Ramband		Root	Water	By grinding	One cup per day	3 days
6. Malaria		*Ataria-ghadi*		Root	Water	By grinding	One cup	3 days
		Malhin tree			Mustered oil	By grinding	—	3 days

1	2	3	4	5	6	7	8	9
		Hing	*Ferula assafoetida*	Gum				
		Gataran	*Caesalpinia crista*	Leaf				
		Neem	*Azadirecta indica*	Stem+ Leaf		By grinding with water	Every morning one cup per day	3-4 days Sour, Chilli, *Udad* Pulse, Spices
		Bel	*Aegel marmelos*	Stem+ Leaf				
		Kali-mirch	*Piper nigrum*	–				
		Tulsi	*Occimum santalum*	Stem+ Leaf				
		Harsanghari	*Nictanthus arbortritis*	Leaves				
		Bhooi neem	*Phyllanthus niruri*	Leaf	Jagery and Honey	Grinding and Making small balls	Two times in a day	3 days Sour Fruit, Brinjal and Beans
		Kalazira						
		Banzeer		Seed				
		Gataran	*Caesalpinia crista*	Leaves				
7. Menstrual Disturbance		*Saal*	*Shorea robusta*	Stem	Sug r or	By	Every	3-4 days
		Kosam	*Scheichera*	Bark	Liq or or	grinding	morning	

1	2	3	4	5	6	7	8	9
			trijuga		Jaggery or water		one cup per day	Sour, Chilli, *Urad* pulse, Spices
		Bhogray		Root				
		Bam		Bark				
		Bahera	*Terminalia bellerica*	Bark				
		Dengarua		Bark				
		Ber	*Ziziphus jujuba*	Bark				
		Katri		Bark				
		Ainthi		Bark				
		Gud-sankri		Root				
		Kurlu		Root and Bark				
		Patthar-chatni		Fruit				
		Chandva		Root				
		Koljamras		Bark				
		Bamri		Root				
		Rakatvirar		Bark				
		Bemchi		Bark				
		Saphed gomchi		Seed				

1	2	3	4	5	6	7	8	9
		Masan jari		Root				
		Dhawai or Salya	*Woodfordia fruticosa*	Flower	Water	By grinding	Every morning one cup per day	1 day
		Dhania		Seed	Water	By grinding	One cup per day	3 days
		Kashyap		Bark	Milk	By grinding	One cup per day	3 days
		Sher		Root	Liquor/water	By grinding	One teaspoon twice a day	3-5 days Sour, *Udad* pulse
		Makra		Root				
		Pharhadda		Bark	Sugar and water	By grinding	One cup per day	3 days
8. Stone		*Chippi*		Root	Sava	By boiling	One cup per day	1 month Sour, Chilli, *Udad* pulse, Spices
		Semar	*Bombax ceiba*	Bark				
		Kirgi		Root	Jaggrey	By grinding	One tablet per day	3 days

1	2	3	4	5	6	7	8	9
		Sher		Tuber		and made Tablet form		
9. Body pain		*Harsanghari*	*Nictanthus arbortritis*	Bark	Water	By grinding.	One cup per day	3 days Sour
		Koria		Bark	Jaggery and water	By grinding.	Half cup per day	Till healing
10. Stomach pain	Phudki	*Black Hen*		Heart	Liquor	By grinding and boiling	One cup per day	3 days
		Dendurwa		Root				
		Phang		Root	Liquor	By grinding	One cup per day	1 day
11. Skin diesease	Chivla rog	*Chivla parsa*		Tuber	Water	By grinding	One cup per day	3 days
		Chind		Tuber				
12. Itching problem		*Semar*	*Bombax ceiba*	Kanta	Mustered oil and Honey	By boiling	Apply in affected areas	Till healing
		Kevchi		Root/ bark				
13. Hydrocele		*Bhengrat*		Tuber	Oil	By	Apply in	3 days

1	2	3	4	5	6	7	8	9
		Kosam	*Scheichera trijuga*	Bark	Oil	grinding	affected areas.	Chilli and spices
14. T.B.		*Malhin*		Bark	Jaggery	By grinding and made tablet form	One tablet per day	7 days
		Nilgiri	*Eucalyptus globulus*	Bark				Sour and cold foods
		Kardhan Mudi		Flower				
15. Mirgi		*Rohina*		Bark	Jaggery	By grinding and made tablet form	One tablet per day	7 days
				–	Camel bone	Grinding with water	One teaspoon twice a day	3 days Sour, *Udad* pulse
16. Cough and cold	Jur	*Tulsi*	*Ocimum sanctum*	Leaf	Honey	Grinding and Mixing	One cup in a day	1 week
		Ginger	*Zinngiber officinale*	Rhi-zome				Sour and Brinjal
		Black pepper	*Piper nigrum*	Rhi-zome				
17. Filaria	Hathipaon	*Black Dhatura*	*Datura stramonium*	Seed	Water	–	Half Spoon	40 days Sour and spicy

1	2	3	4	5	6	7	8	9
								foods
18. Loose motion	Dast	*Garlic*	*Allium sativum*	Bulb	Cold water	—	Five piece two times in a day	2-3 days Hot things
19. Dry Stomach pain		—		—	Fresh urine of Calf		empty stomach	Twice in a day Sour and Cold Thing
20. Wound and Wound with swelling		*Peepal*	*Ficus religiosa*	Root	Hot water	Grinding and Mixing	Apply on wound	One time in a day Sour
21. Vomiting		—		—	Natural *Kapoor* and Sugar	Mixing	Empty stomach	Twice in a day
22. Diabetes		-		—	Urine and bile of Pig	Mixed each other	Three times in a day	One week Sweet things
		Coconut	*Cocus nucifera*	Fruit	Natural *Hing*	Fill 1gm. *Hing* in a complete boll of coconut and use after 15	Twice in a day empty stomach	Two days Sweet things

1	2	3	4	5	6	7	8	9
						days.		
23. Acidity		*Bellgiri*		Outer layer of fruit	Sugar	Boiling with one lt. Water till remains one cup	3 spoon in one day	One week Spicy food
24. Arthritis		*Mathasor*		Root	Water	Grinding and Mixing	One cup daily	One week Sour
		Korya		Root	Water	Grinding and Mixing	Two time Half cup	One week Urad, Bean and Brinjal
25. Bone Fracture		*Harsanghari*	*Nictanthus arbortritis*	Plant (milky)	Hot water	Grinding and Mixing	Tide in damage part. Half cup one time	15 days

Annexure 4 (c)

Medicinal Plant Names—Chhattisgarh

Vernacular Names	*English Names*	*Sanskrit Names*	*Botanical Names*
Aam	Mango tree	*Amra*	*Magifera indica*
Ajmoda	Carom seeds	*Ajmoda*	*Carom roxburghianum*
Akol	Sage leaf	*Ankola*	*Alangium lamarckii*
Akvan	Madar	*Ark*	*Calotropis procera*
Amarvel	Giant Dodder	*Amarvel*	*Cuscuta reflexa*
Afim	Opium Poppy	*Ahiphen*	*Papaver somniferum*
Asagandh	Winter cherry	*Ashwagandha*	*Withania somnifera*
Babul	*Babul*a tree, Indian Gum tree	*Babbula*	*Acaacia arabica*
Bahera	Belleric Myrobalan	*Bibhitak*	*Terminalia bellerica*
Banjir	Holy Basil	*Ajaka*	*Occimum gratissimum*
Bakayan	Melia azadirecta	*Mahanimb*	*Beed tree*
Ber	Ziziphus	*Badar*	*Ziziphus jujula*
Bhatkataiyya	Indian Nightshade	*Kantakari*	*Solanum indicum*
Bhindi	Orka/Lady finger	*Bhindika*	*Abelmoschus esculentus*
Bhui Nimb	Stone breaker	*Bhumyamalaki*	*Phyllanthus niruri*
Chitavar	Leadwort	*Chitrak*	*Plumbago zeylanica*
Chiraiyata	Green Chirayata	*Kalmegh*	*Andrographis*

Vernacular Names	*English Names*	*Sanskrit Names*	*Botanical Names*
			paniculata
Dantul			
Dhatura	Thorn apple	*Kanak*	*Datura alba*
Galgala	Yellow Flowered Cotton Tree	*Girimallika*	*Cochlospermum gossypium*
Gengrua	Rosselle, Red Sorrel	*Ambasthaki*	*Hibiscus sabdariffa*
Dahiman (Shikari)	Dayyad	—	*Cordia macleodi*
Dhavai	Fireflame bush	*Dhataki*	*Woodfordia fruticosa*
Dhania	Coriander	*Dhanyak*	*Cooriander sativum*
Gataran	Fever Nut	*Latakaranj*	*Caesalpinia rista*
Gomachi	Crab's Eye	*Gunja*	*Abrus precotaria*
Guruch	Tinospora	*Guduchi*	*Tinospora cordifolia*
Tinpatia	Indian Sorrel	*Changeri*	*Oxalis corniculata*
Tinsa	Sandan	*Tinish*	*Oogenia dalbergioides*
Jimikand	Elephant's foot	*Suran, Arshognya*	*Amorphophallus campanulatus*
Jamun	Jambol	*Jambu*	*Syzygium cumin/ Eugenia jambolana*
Singhari	Water Caltrops/ Indian Water Chest Nut	*Shrungatak*	*Trapa bi-spinosa*
Sal	Sal Tree	*Agnivallabha, Ashwakarna*	*Shorea robusta*
Satavar	Asparagus	*Shatavari*	*Aspareagus racemosus*
Saphed Musali	Land Calotrops	*Shweta Musali*	*Cholophytum tuberosa*
Semar	Red Silk Cotton tree	*Shalmali*	*Bombax ceiba*
Sonth	Dry Ginger	*Sunth*	*Zingiber officicnale*
Kans	Sugar Cane	*Ekshvaku*	*Sachharum*

Vernacular Names	*English Names*	*Sanskrit Names*	*Botanical Names*
			spontanum
Kala Dhatura	Black Datura	*Krushna Dhattur*	*Datura stramonium*
Kala Jeera	Krishna Jeera	*Black Cumin*	*Bunium persicum*
Kali Mirch	Black Pepper	*Marich*	*Piper nigrum*
Katai	Febrifuge plant	*Kantakari*	*Solanum xanthocarpum*
Katari	Purging nut	*Danti*	*Jatropa curcas*
Koraiyya	Kurchi, Conessi	*Kutaj*	*Holarrhena antidysentrica*
Kosam	Kusum, Lace tree	*Koshamra*	*Scheichera trigjuga*
Lahsun	Garlic	*Rason*	*Allium sativum*
Lavki	Bottle Gourd	*Alabu*	*Lagenaria scieraria*
Neem	Margosa tree	*Nimb*	*Azadirecta indica*
Madar	Crown Plant	*Mandar*	*Calatropis gigantean*
Mahua	Indian Butter Tree	*Madhuk*	*Madhuka indica*
Mirch	Red Pepper	*Katuvira*	*Capsicum annum*
Ganja	Marijuana	*Bhanga*	*Canabis sativa*
Galagal	Yellow flowered cotton tree	*Girishalmalika*	*Cochlospermum gossypium*
Gatarun	Fever nut	*Lata Karanj*	*Caesalpinia crista*
Gengrua	Roselle	*Ambasthaki*	*Hibiscus sabdariffa*
Gomachi	Jequirity seed	*Gunja*	*abrus precatorius*
Harsinghari	Night-flowering Jasmine	*Parijatak*	*Nictanthus arbortritis*
Hing	Asafetida	*Hingu*	*Ferula assafoetida*
Indraban	Bitter snake-gourd	*Indravaruni*	*Trichosanthes tricuspidata*
Pepper	Indian long pepper	*Pippali*	*Piper longum*
Tinpatiyan	Indian Sorrel	*Changeri*	*Oxalis corniculata*

Annexure 5 (a)

Home Remedies: Tribal Blocks—Maharashtra

Home Remedy: Herbs

Community know following plants and how to use to treat ailments at home: (Etapalli : District Gadchiroli) Sawar sal, Kumabhai sal, Kuda, Shatavari, Hirada, Behada, Jambol, Mugna, Panfuti, Gul neeli, Nagveli, Vagoti, rakta shehda, Kudabi, Mekad, Wild Onion, Peddma, Alantu, Tentu, Papaya, Saphed Musali, Vavding, Murud sheng, Todambi, bile of fish, Ud.

Tribal groups from Etapalli use Mashrooms, Matalu (a type of *kand*), fish.

Tribal Community (Mokhada, District Palghar)

Tribal families know the identification and use of following herbs:

Awala, Pachar Kanda, Behada, Nirgundi, Hirda, Murud sheng, Moh, Arjun, Panfuti, Amba, Shevga, Hadsandhi, Korphad, Shatavari, Kadunimb, Papai, Fanas, Palas, Sid Muli, Saval sal Bhui Awala, Bahava, Koshimbi, Lemon (Linmbu), Kadi Patta, Karanj, Chinch, Bor, Kusar Ranshevga, Phangala, Chafa, Aerand, Mehandi, Sagargota, Bhuskut, Ambadi, Kuyari, Sagvani bee, Harali kand, Umber sal, Jambhul sal.

At house level people know about following herbs: (Rajur, Akole: District A'nagar)

Hirda, Arjun, Tantani, Dhotara, Shatavari, Ran kanda, Kallavi, White Hibiscus, Kolsuna, Lemon, Turmaric, Aekadicha pala, Raktohin, Pudina, Dry ginger, Aloe vera, Dry Coriander, Jaggery, Castor (Aerand), Indian flame tree (Palas), Chtrak, Aliv, Sagrgota, Nagveli, Murud sheng, Gunja pala, Awala, Ritha, Bharangi, Bahava.

Kitchen Garden Herbs: (Zari Zamni, District Yavatmal)

Margosa, Kate Sawar, Adulsa, Raktarohada, Maharukh, Jambhul, Sagargota, Vaghati, Bhui Nimb, Turmaric, Tulasi, Shevga, Lasun, Pimperkhed, Palas these are some herb which villagers have in their kitchen garden and farms and know the use of them.

People use Following Herbs: (Akkalkuva, District Nandurbar)

Margosa, Dendva, Jambol, Asparagus, Pepper, Cordifolia, Rakta Rohda, Nakhyo, Tohgoval, Bihrav, Bodo oohav, Tvara Motho.

People has Knowledge about Following Herbs: (Jawhar, District Palghar)

Hirda, Behada, Awala, Onion, Castor, Lemon, Margosa, Karanj oil, Adulasa, Kumbhai, Kuda, Jambl, Ficus tree, Black catechue, Five leave chaste, Butter tree, Palas, Aspparagus, Ginger, Bahva, Arjun, Raktarohij, Saphed Musali.

Annexure 5 (b) (i)

Plants/Herbs used by Vaidus—Maharashtra

Commonly used Herbs by Vaidus (Etapalli, District Gadchiroli)

Kadunimb, Bhui Nemb, Hirda, Behada, Bala, Nirgudi, Gulvel, Shatavari, Bahava, Salai, Palas, Tembaruche, Jambhul, Umbar, Kavath, Tonbi, Moh, Pandhara Dhotara, Pivala Dhotra, Hira Mohiti, Bhui Palas, Babhali, Nagveli, Saphed Ark, Khavaskhuri, Jangali Halad, Ran Amba, Chinch, Palas, Rakt Behada, Nilgiri, Bor, Tulas, Gavti chaha, Kumbhai, Akkalkara, Bahva, Shatavari, Kuda, Vad, Taet.

They use these medicines in the form of *churn* (powder), *Swaras* (juice), *lep* (Local Application).

Vaidu: (Mokhada, District Palghar)

Herbs used by all vaidu are Hirda, Behada, Ranbhendi, Karanj, Palas, Kuda, Shid, Bahava, Tentu, Sag, Jambhul, Roots of Shatavari, Pehashichi sal, Barora mul, Peru Muli, Mirachi, Galachi Sal, Aerand, Rankanda.

Vaidu Knows Following Herbs (Rajur, Akole, District A'nagar)

Shatavari, Kusar, Awala, Jambhul, Kala kua, Amba, Behada, Anantmul, Hirda, Aerand, Bhuskut, Chafa, Kamal, Jatashankar, Tambadi ambi, Lal Gunja, Kumbha, Palas, Ran Kavali, Jeshtmadh, Arjun, Suran, Saphed Musali, Kali Musali, Malkangoni, Nagarmotha, Bilayat, Dhotra, Kolsuna, Ambad

Aedangi, Adulsa, Dhayati, Lala Kesar, Pandhara Budhaval, Pamdhara Ladga, Sawar, Bor, Fangala, Murud sheng.

Vaidu: (Dhadgaon, District Nandurbar)

Some of the Names of Herbs which Vaidu Knows

Sagargota, Jirmya, Vagh nakhya, Rakohida, Germal, Mirchikand, Ukhivala, Gungala, Kadu nimb, Kuda, Kumbha, Bola, Jmabhul, Hariyo, Bhugali, Modalo, Palas, Moricha, Ath hakala, Limbu.

Vaidu has Knowledge about following Herbs (Zari zamni, District Yavatmal)

Adulsa, Shatavari, Tulas, Bhui Nimb, Rohini, Palas, Bel, Behada, Nilgiri, Awala, Vath, Moh, Nagfeni, Ashwagandha, Nimb, Kate savari, Rui, Khadunchkarta, Sag, Bahva, Nilgiri, Amba, Khair, Vad, Jambhul, Kesa.

Vaidu (Akkalkuva, District Nandurbar)

Commonly used herbs by vaidus are Five leaves chaste, Asparagus, Guggul, Cordifolia, Margosa, Kuda, Rakta rohada etc.

Vaidus can Identify Following Herbs: (Jawhar, District Palghar)

Moh, Kharshing, Hirda, Behada, Palsa, Kahdol, Bahava, Khumbhai, Savar, Sonchafa, Murud sheng, Nirgundi, Adulsa, Pandhari Gunj, Lala Gunj, Hadmodi, Umbar, Khair, Karnaj, Kuda.

Vaidu: (Dharni, District Amravati)

Following herb are collected by Vidus from Jangle-Bokoch: Buti, Margosa, Maethkal, Jad kumbhi, outer covering of bark of Jambol tree and bel, flowers of Indian Butter tree, leaves of five chaste, outer covering of bark of Nila Kata, Saphed Akva, Dev Kapus, Saphed plus, Bhui Rengali.

Vaidu uses Panchang—flower, leaves, outer covering of bark of tree, root, fruit of medicinal herbs. These can be given in different forms like juice, *lep*, powder etc.

Annexure 5 (b) (ii)

Diseases Treated by Vaidus—Maharashtra

Local Vaidus Treat following Diseases: (Mokhada, District Palghar)

Jaundice, gynecological problems, worms infestation, itching and skin diseases, tumours on neck, piles, snake bite, bodyache, Diarrhoea, bone fracture. They also knew the concepts like Nagali, Rice and Dal easy to digest.

Pregnant ladies are advised not to eat Papaya, Jack fruit, Ground Nuts.

In post partum period 5 days after delivery new mothers advised to eat Nagali or Varai chi Pej. Brinjal, Mata, Pawata are not given in post partum period and advised to have Asparagus roots for breast milk enhancement.

Vaidu Treats following Conditions: (Rajur, Akole: District A'nagar)

Piles, Joint pain, Bruising, Wound, Fever, Diarrhoea, Rickets, Malnutrition, Ring worm, Cancer, Puncture wound, Paralysis, Jaundice, Scorpion bite, Stomachache, Migraine, Renal stones, Gynaecological problems, Toothache, Diabetes, Veterinary diseases.

Form of medicine decided by vaidu depending upon the type of disease (Dhadgaon, Diarrhea Nandurbar)

Common diseases treated by Vaidu—Convulsions, Edema of limbs, Lower backache, Fever, Stomachache after Delivery.

Piles, fever, diarrhoea are the common diseases treated by Vaidus.

Commonly Treated Conditions: (Akkalkuva, District Nandurbar)

Diarrhoea, Vomiting, Lower backache, Backache, Cough, Cold.

Commonly Treated Conditions by Vaidu: (Jawhar, District Palghar)

Insufficient breast milk, infertility, joint pain, jaundice, urinary track infection, paediatric illnesses, scorpion bite, snake bite, skin diseases, tomour in abdomen, nausea.

Commonly treated conditions by Vaidu (Dharni, District Amravati)

Infertility, jaundice, headache, pain in abdomen.

Annexure 5 (b) (iii)

Vaidu Remedies, Tribal Blocks–Maharashtra

Sl. No.	*Symptom*	*Districts (Tribal Blocks)*						
		Palghar	*Raigad*	*Nandurbar*	*A'nagar*	*Yavatmal*	*Amravati*	*Gadchiroli*
		Material Used						
1	2	3	4	5	6	7	8	9
1.	Cough	Bhabhali, Adulsa, Korfad, Ava, Halad, Borichi sal, Kapur, Khobarel tel.	Adulsa, —Tulsi, Adulsa	Outer covering of bark of Rona crushed in water. —Ginger, gargling by turmeric and	Young black chebulei + Honey. —Young Chebulei + Honey, Winter	Ginger, Adulsa. —Flower of calatropis given with the juice of Nagveli, Tulas,	Ginger, Honey —Smoke of powder of Bajara, Garlic, Hinger + Honey, Jaggery +	Ginger, Black Pepper, Holy Basil leaves, Carom Seeds, Black chebuli (Hirda), Sitopaladi churn, Indian

1	2	3	4	5	6	7	8	9
		Hirda, Outer covering of bark of Bori, Adulsa		salt water, Movasi root	cherry, Black Pepper, Decoction of dry ginger, turmeric powder + powder of cloves + Black pepper + Honey	Adulsa	Turmaric powder	licorice (Yashti-madhu) + Indian Gooseberry (Awala)
2.	Cold	Holy Basil leaves, Jagerry + Onion, Carom seeds. Tulasi, Ginger	Carom seeds. —Vapour	Tulasi	Smoke of Bajra powder, Carom seeds, Garlic + Salt		Ginger, Honey —Vapour	Holy Basil leaves, Lemon Grass, Turmeric powder
3.	Fever	Decoction of Chirette sticks	Tulasi, Decoction of Pepper		Juice of Holy Basil and Mint	Bhui Nimb, Tulasi. —Lavang,	Tulasi, Kuda seed	Decoction of Chirette sticks (Chiraita)

1	2	3	4	5	6	7	8	9
		(Papada) —Tulasi —Tulasi, Kuda seed			leaves	Dry Ginger, Black Pepper, decoction of Pepper, decoction of Bhui Nimb, Margosa		
4.	Diarrhoea	Juice of Fangala			Root of Chitrak given by crushing	Lemon Drink. —Sweat Sago soup, savar sal, Margosa,	Salt, lemon, water drink —Salt+ lemon + water drink, Yogurt + sugar	Sugar and salt dissolved in water, Outer covering of bark of Jejube (Bor)
5.	Vomiting			Decoction of Turmeric	Aloe vera, Murud sheng, Salt + Sugar+ Lemon (Drink)	Lemon drink		Drink made up of Lemon
6.	Headache			Root of Huja crushed in	Black salt + Garlic,	Garlic	Garlic juice in nose	Black tea, Indian

1	2	3	4	5	6	7	8	9
				water	Garlic, Chitrak, Local application of lime			Gooseberry (Awala), Clarified Butter
7.	Bodyache			Dev Halad	Outer covering of bark of Arjun boiled in water and used for hot fomentation, lcally apply oil of DP	Five leave chaste, Takala, leaves of Melsing		Bath taken with decoction of Five Leave Chaste (Nirgundi) leaves
8.	Lower Backache	Nirgudi Oil, Sagargota Bee —Nirgunn-di tel	Leaves of Nirgundi				Mustard oil massage, Massage with kerosene	Ginger, Honey, Oil made up of Heart leaf Sida or Flannel weed (Bala)

1	2	3	4	5	6	7	8	9
9.	Stomachache	Murud Sheng, Pulp of Aloe vera, Soda, Water of Ambadi. —Outer covering of bark of Kumbai	Leaves of Margosa leaves, Tulas, Aloe vera, Turmeric powder, Cordifolia, Murud sheng, lemon grass	Kodvacha pala	Decoction of eucalyptus leaves, dry ginger + dry coriander + jaggery+ sagargota			Ashes from Chulha, Salt, Soil, Carom seeds, Black salt, Local application of Asafetida (*Hing*) on area surrounding umbilicus
10.	Worms	Pachar Onion, Wild Onion, Seed of Drum stick	Seed of Indian Flame tree, Mirsing, juice of leaves of Bamboo tree	Root of Dati	Drum stick seed, powder of sagargota seed	Crushed leaves of Margosa tree		Indian Flame tree (*Palash*) seed, Kudabi, Pulp of Drum Stick or Purging Cassia (*Bahava*)
11.	Skin Disease	Juice of Margosa leaves	Leaves of Margosa tree	Root of Sida	Extract of calotropis	Cow's urine	Leaves of Waja, Utaran vel	Margosa (*Kadunimb*)

1	2	3	4	5	6	7	8	9
		(*Kadu* nimb)						
12.	Weakness			Saphed Mushali				Awala, Khadisakhar
13.	Wound	Margosa leaves. —Turmeric powder	Juice of Leaves of Fangala	Lag Mathi	Leaves of Fangulna Leaves of Margosa, Tantani	Leaves of Khandu-chkar	Aloe vera pulp	Turmeric, outer covering of bark of Mulberry (*Tendu*), leaves of Kambarmodi
14.	Bone Fracture	Hadsandhi		Lothra decoction				Cordifolia (*Gulvel*), Wild Mango
15.	Jaundice	Outer covering of bark of Mango tree, Cow's Urine (*Gomutra*),	Juice of Cordifolia leaves, extract of Castor and calotropis tree	Crab, Juice of sugar cane	Juice of leaves of Thorn apple + Juice of leaves of Castor +		Juice of Castor leaves twice a day	Gripe Weed (*Bhui Awala*), Outer covering of bark of Asoka tree

1	2	3	4	5	6	7	8	9
		Lemon, Sugar, Salt			Milk			
16.	Wight gain in children							Young roots of Mulberry (*Tendu*), outer covering of Kujar weed
17.	For easy and safe delivery				Decoction of Black Pepper			Receptacle (*deth*) of Indian Butter tree (*Moh*)
18.	Joint Pain	Oil of Five leaves Chaste (*Nirgundi*)		Mirchi kand	Hot fomentation by Nir-gundi, root of Chitrak, Local appli-cation	Hot fomentation by Nirgundi leaves —Leaves of Drumstick		
19.	Limb (Hand and Feet) Pain				Hot fomen-tation by Five Leaves			

1	2	3	4	5	6	7	8	9
					Chaste			
20.	Gynecological problems	Outer covering of Sal and Ficus tree, flower of Indian flame tree		Root of Jivil Ukhavil	Powder of flower of Indian flame tree, flower of white hibscus		Juice of leaves of Margosa tree	
21.	Unconsciousness		Onion	Onion put near nose. - Onion	Onion put near nose	Onion	Onion	
22.	Insufficient breast milk						Flowers of Indian butter tree + Jaggery + Musali powder + Decoction of Asparagus, Flowers of Indian butter tree roasted in *Ghee* + tea	

1	2	3	4	5	6	7	8	9
							made up of jaggery.	
23.	Edema		Raktarohida					
24.	Scorpion bite				Vekhand			
25.	Nausea				Jambhul kurudu			

Annexure 5 (c)

Medicinal Plant Names—Maharashtra

Sl. No.	*Vernacular Name*	*English Name*	*Hindi Name*	*Sanskrit Name*	*Botanical Name*
1.	*Aale*	Ginger	Adrak	*Ardrak*	*Zingiberofficinale*
2.	*Aerand*	Castor oil plant	Aerand	*Erand*	*Rcinuscommunis*
3.	*Ahaliv*	Common cress, Garden cress	Akalam, Candsur	*Ahaleev, Bhadra, Chandrica*	*Lepidiumsativum*
4.	*Amba*	Mango	Aam	*Amra*	*Mangiferaindica*
5.	*Ambadi*	Kenaf leaves	Patasan	*Machika*	*Hibiscus cannabinus/sabdariffa*
6.	*Anantmul*	Indian sarsaparilla	Anantmul	*Sariva*	*Hemidesmusindicus*

Sl. No.	Vernacular Name	English Name	Hindi Name	Sanskrit Name	Botanical Name
7.	*Ark*	Madar	Aak	*Ark*	*Caotropisprocera*
8.	*Ashwagandha*	Winter cherry	Asagandh	*Ashwagandha*	*Withaniasomnifera*
9.	*Ashok*	False Ashoka Tree	Ashok	*Ashok*	*Saracaasoka*
10.	*Awala*	Indian gooseberry	Awala	*Amalaki*	*Phyllanthusembellica*
11.	*Bahva*	Canafistula, Golden shower	Amaltas	*Argvadh*	*Cassia fistula*
12.	*Behada*	Belericmyrobolan	Behra	*Bidhitak, Aksha*	*Terminalia belerica*
13.	*Bhuiawala*	Stone Breaker	Bhuiamala	*Bhumyamlaki*	*Phyllanthusniruri*
14.	*Bhui Nimb*	King of bitters, Green Chirayta	Kalmegh	*Mahatikta, Kalmegh*	*Andrographispanniculata*
15.	*Bhui Rengali*	Wild Egg Plant	Kateli, Katai	*Kantakari*	*Solanumxanthocarpum*
16.	*Bor*	Jejube	Ber	*Badar*	*Ziziphusmauritiana*
17.	*Chitrak*	Lead wort	Cheeta	*Chitrak, Agni*	*Plumbagzeylanica*
18.	*Chinch*	Tamrind	Emali	*Amlika*	*Tamarindusindica*
19.	*Dhayati*	Fire flame bush	Dahwai	*Dhataki*	*Woodfordiafuiticosa*
20.	*Dudhali*	Semi erect Euphorbia	Chotidudhi	*Dughadhika*	*Euphorbia thymifolia*
21.	*Dudhkand*	Milky Yam	Vidari	*KshirVidari*	*Ipomeadigita*
22.	*Dhotra*	Thorn Apple	Dhatura	*Dhattur*	*Daturametel*
23.	*Fanas*	Jackfruit	Katahal	*Panas*	*Artocarpusheterophyllus*

Sl. No.	*Vernacular Name*	*English Name*	*Hindi Name*	*Sanskrit Name*	*Botanical Name*
24.	*Phangul*	Vegetable gourd	Torai	*TiktaKoshataki, Jalini*	*Luffaacutangula*
25.	*Gulvel*	Cordifolia	Gulbel	*Guduchi*	*Tinosporacordifolia*
26.	*Hadaki*	Indian snakeroot	Chota Chand, Dhawalbarua, Pagalkibuti	*Sarpagandha*	*Raufoliaserpentina*
27.	*Hadasandhi*	Devil's Backbone	Hadjot	*Asthisamharak*	*Cissusquadrangularis*
28.	*Hing*	Asafoetida, Devil's dung	Hing	*Hingu*	*Ferula asafetida*
29.	*Hirda*	Myrobalan, Chebulicmyobalan	Harad	*Haritaki*	*Terminalia Chebula*
30.	*Jambhul*	Jambol	Jamun	*Jambu*	*Syzygium cumin/Eugenia jambolana*
31.	*Jeshtamadh*	Indian licorice	Mulethi	*Yastimadhu*	*Glycyrrhizaglabera*
32.	*Kali Kavali*	Indian sarsapanila	Anantmul	*KrushnaSariva*	*Hemidesmusindicus*
33.	*Kambarmodi*	Coat Buttons	Ghamara, Khal muriya	*Jayantiveda*	*Tridexprocumbance*
34.	*Kanda*	Onion	Pyas	*Palandu*	*Aliumcepa*
35.	*Kadunimb*	Margosa plant	Neem	*Nimba*	*Azadirectaindica*
36.	*Khair*	Black Catechu	Kathha	*Gayatri*	*Acasia catechu*

Sl. No.	Vernacular Name	English Name	Hindi Name	Sanskrit Name	Botanical Name
37.	*Kohla*	Ground Melon ash pumkin	Kohla	*Kushmanda*	*Cucurbitahispida*
38.	*Kuda, Kuda bee*	Bitter Oleander, Dysentery Rose Bay	KadvaIndrajav	*Kutaj*	*Holerrhenaantidysentrica*
39.	*Kumbhai*	Wild Guava, Ceylon Oak, Patana Oak	Kumbhi	*Kumbhi*	*Coreyaarborea*
40.	*Kusar*	Wild Jasmine	Banamallika	*Vanmallika, Ashota*	*Jasminumangustifolium*
41.	*Lal Gunja*	Red Coral Bead Vine	Ghungachi	*Rakta Gunja*	*Abrusprecatorius*
42.	*Lavang*	Clove	Laung	*Lavang, Devkusum*	*Syzygiumaromaticum*
43.	*Limbu*	Lemon	Nimbu	*Nimbuk*	*Citrus aurantifolia*
44.	*Maithfal*	Emetic nut	Mainfal	*Madanfal*	*Randiadumetorum*
45.	*Matalu (Dukkar Kand)*	Air Potato	Jimikand	*Varahi*	*Discoeabulbifera*
46.	*Mehandi*	Henna	Mahandi	*Madayantica*	*Lowsoniainermis*
47.	*Mire*	Black pepper	Kali mirch	*Marich*	*Piper nigrum*
48.	*Moh*	Indian Butter tree	Mahua	*Madhuka*	*Madhucaindica*
49.	*Nagfeni*	Prickly Pear	Nagfana	*Snuhi*	*Opuntiadillenii*
50.	*Nagveli*	Betel Leaves	Pan Patta	*Tambulpatra*	*Piper bitel*
51.	*Nilgiri*	Eucalyptus tree	Nilgiri	*Tailpatra, Sugandhpatra*	*Eucallyptus globules*

Sl. No.	Vernacular Name	English Name	Hindi Name	Sanskrit Name	Botanical Name
52.	*Nirgundi*	Five/Three leaves cheste	Nirgundi	*Nirgundi, Shefali*	*VitexNigundo*
53.	*Ova*	Carom seeds	Ajwain	*Ajmoda*	*Carumroxburghiianum*
54.	*Pandharigunj*	White Coral Bead Vine	Ghungachi	*Shweta Gunja*	*Abrusprecatorius*
55.	*Papai*	Papaya	Papita	*Madhukarkati*	*Carica papaya*
56.	*Palas*	Indian Flame tree	Palas	*Palas*	*Butea monosperma*
57.	*Panfuti*	Miracle life, Wonder of life	Amar poi	*Parnabij*	*Bryophyllumpinnatum*
58.	*Rankanda*	Milk and Wine Lily	Sudarshan	*Madhuparnika*	*Crinum latifolium*
59.	*Ran kavali*	Country sarsaparila	Anantmul	*Sariva*	*Hemidesmuindicus*
60.	*Ritha*	Soap nut	Ritha	*Arishtak*	*Sapindustrifoliatus*
61.	*Rohini*	Hellebore	Kutaki	*Katuka, Katurohini*	*Picrorhizakurroa*
62.	*Sabudana*	Sago	Shakarkand	*Tarukanda, Kalpakand*	*Manihotesculenta*
63.	*Sag*	Teak	Saigun	*Saka*	*Tectonagrandis*
64.	*Sagargota*	Fever nut	Kantakarej	*LataKaranj*	*Caesalpinia crista*
65.	*Satavar*	Indian Asparagus, Hundred Root	Satavar	*Shatavari*	*Asparagus racemosa*
66.	*Savar*	Silk Cotton Tree	Semar	*Shalmali*	*Salmaliamalbarica*
67.	*Sawar*	Silk cotton tree	Semar	*Shalmali*	*Bombaxceiba*
68.	*Shevaga*	Drumstick	Munaga	*Shigru*	*Moringaoleifera*

Sl. No.	Vernacular Name	English Name	Hindi Name	Sanskrit Name	Botanical Name
69.	*Shid/Sid*	Bidi leaf tree	Jhinjheri	*Yugmapatra tree*	*Bauhinia racemosa*
70.	*Takal*	Sickelsenna	Charota	*Chakramurd*	*Cassia to:a*
71.	*Tantani*	Lantana	Ran Munia	*Chaturangi, Vanacchedi*	*Lantana camara*
72.	*Tendu*	White mulberry	Shahtoot	*Tud*	*Morus alba*
73.	*Til*	Sesame seed plant	Til	*Til*	*Sisamumindicum*
74.	*Ud*	Dhup tree	Kala dammer	*Dhupvruksha, Raladhup*	*Canariumstrictum*
75.	*Utran*	Trellis –Vine	Utran, Sagovani	*Visanika, Uttarmavini, Kurutakah*	*Pergulariadaemia*
76.	*Vad*	Banyan tree	Bargad	*Vatvruksha*	*Ficusbenghalensis*
77.	*Vaghnakhya*	Tiger's claw, Devil's claw	Ulatkanta	*Kaknasa*	*Martyniaannua*

REFERENCES

Basham, A.L., 1954, *The Wonder that was India*, Grove Press, New York.

Bhat, H.K. Joshi, P.C. Vijayendra, B.R. (ed) 2013: *Explorations in Indian Medical Anthropology* (Vol. I & II), Concept Publishing Co. (P) Ltd., New Delhi.

Department of AYUSH, 1999: *An Appraisal of Tribal Folk Medicine*, CCRAS, New Delhi.

Department of AYUSH, 2003: *Handbook of Common Remedies in Unani System of Medicine*, CCRUS, New Delhi.

Department of AYUSH, 2005: *Handbook of Domestic Medicine and Common Ayurvedic Medicine*, CCRAS, New Delhi.

Department of AYUSH, 2006: *AYUSH Task Force Report for Eleventh Five Year Plan*, Government of India, New Delhi.

Department of AYUSH, 2011: *AYUSH in India 2010*, New Delhi.

Department of Health and Family Welfare, 2002: *National ISM&H Policy*, Government of India, New Delhi.

Department of Health and Family Welfare, 2002, *National Health Policy*, Government of India, New Delhi.

Dube, S.C., 1958, *India's Changing Villages*, Routledge.

Foster, G.M., Anderson, B.G. 1978, *Medical Anthropology*, John Wiley & Sons, New York.

Leslie, Charles (ed.) 1976, *Asian Medical Systems: A Comparative Study*, University of California Press, Berkeley.

Leslie Charles (ed.) 1980, *Social Science and Medicine* 14 B (4), Special Issue: Medical Pluralism: Proceedings of Pune Symposium on Medical Anthropology, Pergamon Press.

Mutatkar, R.K., Danda, Ajit K., Bhatt, Vikas (ed.): 2010, *Studies on Bio-Medical Anthropology*, INCAA, Jhargram and IGRMS, Bhopal.

Mutatkar R.K., 2013, *Review article on Status of Indian Medicine and Folk Healing*, Part 2 by Shailaja Chandra in J-AIM, 4(3) pp. 184-185.

Mutatkar, Kalpana, 2013, Practicing Medical Anthropology: Addressing Malnutrition among Tribal Children in Bhat, *et al.* (ed.)

Explorations in Indian Medical Anthropology, (Vol. II) Concept Publishing Co. (P) Ltd., New Delhi.

NHSRC Report by Ritu Priya and Shweta, A.S., 2010, *Status and Role of AYUSH and Local Health Traditions* under NRHM, New Delhi.

Padam Singh *et al.*, 2005, Utilisation of Indigenous Systems of Medicine and Homeopathy in India, *Indian J. Med.* Res, August, pp. 137-142, ICMR, New Delhi

Pandit, C.G., 1982, *My World of Preventive Medicine,* ICMR, New Delhi.

Planning Commission, 2006, *AYUSH Report of Steering Committee for 11th Five Year Plan,* (2007-2012), Government of India, New Delhi.

Planning Commission, 2006, *Steering Committee Working Group on AYUSH in Public Health,* Government of India, New Delhi.

Planning Commission, 2011, *AYUSH Report of Steering Committee for 12th Five Year Plan* (2012-2017), Government of India, New Delhi.

Redfield, Robert, 1962, Human Nature and the Study of Society, University of Chicago Press, Chicago.

SEDEM Report by Arun Srivastava, 2010, *Assessment of AYUSH in Rajasthan after Mainstreaming,* New Delhi.

Shailaja Chandra, 2011, *Status of Indian Medicine and Folk Healing,* Pt. 1, Department of AYUSH, Government of India.

Shailaja Chandra, 2013, *Status of Indian Medicine and Folk Healing,* Pt. 2, Department of AYUSH, Government of India.

Vaidya, A.B., Antarkar, D.S., 1981, The use of scientifically valid herbs and plants in primary health care, *Indian Journal of Medical Research,* pp. 79-86, ICMR, New Delhi.

WHO, 1983, *Traditional Medicine and Health Care Coverage* (ed.) by Bannerman, *et al.*, Geneva.

WHO, 2002, *WHO Traditional Medicine Strategy 2002-2005,* Geneva.

INDEX